We're All In This Together

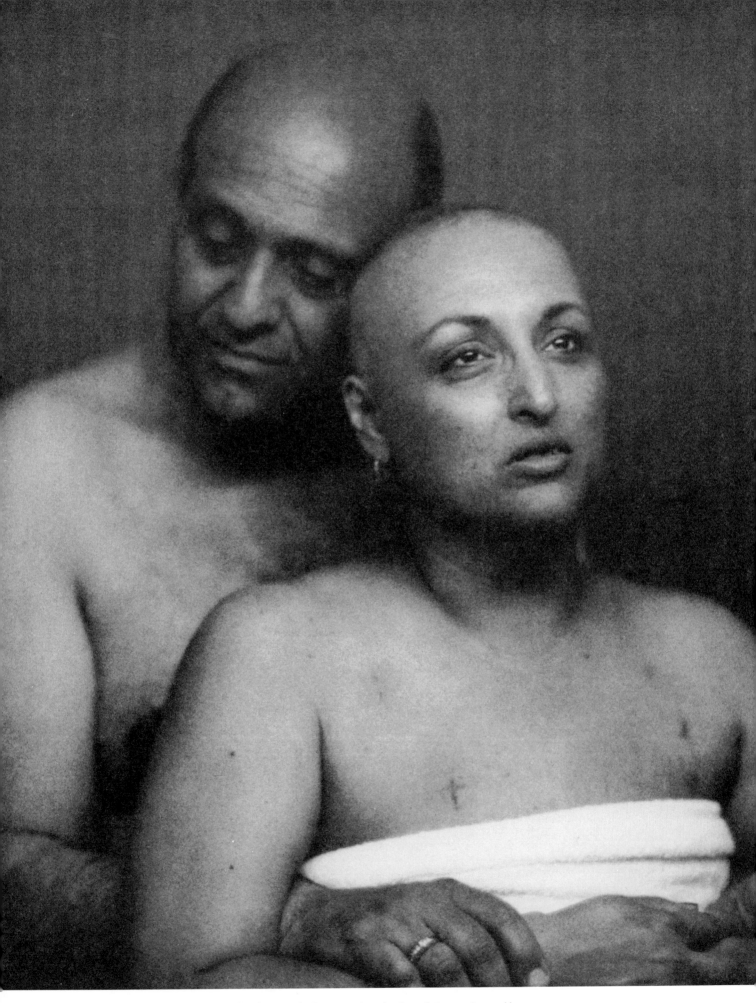

Jerry and Fran Lenzo looking into the mirror of their hotel room in the Poconos, where they have their annual second honeymoon.

We're All In This Together

Families Facing Breast Cancer

by Irene Virag

photographs by Erica Berger

Newsday

ANDREWS AND McMEEL

A Universal Press Syndicate Company

Kansas City

Additional copies of this book may be ordered by calling (800) 642-6480.

Library of Congress Cataloging-in-Publication Data
Virag, Irene.
    We're all in this together : families facing breast cancer / by
Irene Virag ; photographs by Erica Berger.
        p.   cm.
    ISBN 0-8362-7050-9
    1. Breast—Cancer—Case studies.   2. Breast—Cancer—Patients—
—Family relationships.   I. Title.
RC280.B8V57   1995
362.1'9699449—dc20   94-44751
                                                        CIP

Book design: Barrie Maguire
Cover photographs: Erica Berger
Black and white prints: Mike Amoruso/Lexington Labs

For Harvey Aronson,
the best of husbands and always the best of editors.

For Samuel and Susan Berger

ACKNOWLEDGMENTS

We'd like to thank our *Newsday* editors on this project: Bob Tiernan, Charlotte Hall, Howard Schneider, Ken Irby, James Dooley.

We also appreciate the help of Rosemarie Ampela of North Shore University Hospital, Gail Probst of Huntington Hospital and Dr. Karen Kostroff of Long Island Jewish Hospital.

And above all, we're grateful to the brave women who made this book possible—as well as their families and friends.

Contents

Prologue

My editors at *Newsday* are fond of saying that I write about the human condition. This has a nice ring but to me it's always seemed like another euphemism for tragedy. During my thirteen years at *Newsday*, I've been asked to give faces to homelessness and poverty and voices to grief and old age. I've written about the sandwich generation squeezed between the needs of grown children and their own aging parents. I've written about a teenage girl trapped in the mourning and memory of a twin sister lost in the instant carnage of an auto accident and about a young couple who would never stop grieving for the infant son killed in a plane crash they had survived. I've written about Amerasian youngsters yearning for their lost heritage in the land of their fathers—the GIs who had abandoned them to lives as outcasts on the streets of Vietnam. And I spent a year telling the story of a young divorced mother from middle-class suburbia fighting to pull herself out of welfare.

It would be professional to say that these things never touched me—journalists are supposed to stay outside their stories. The old objectivity line. Death and despair, I'd tell anyone who asked, that's my beat. We're reporters. Tears are strictly for the people we chronicle.

But there came a point when I asked my editor to please, oh please, give me an assignment where the people I wrote about didn't cry when I interviewed them. The tears were contagious after all—I just kept them from showing. The tears caught at the edges of my soul when a missing three-year-old was found in the surf where she had been drowned by her drug-addicted mother. They welled up when I watched a priest hold a mass for his murdered mother. They gathered when an Amerasian girl danced in the first snow she had ever seen and cried out "I'm home" to the falling flakes.

Of course, I had an out. I knew intellectually that things like murder and poverty were within the realm of possibility in my own life but viscerally I didn't think they could ever happen to me. I couldn't say that when the assignment was breast cancer.

Even though I had never known anyone with breast cancer I was like every women on Long Island, where the disease is dramatically evident. I was like every women in America. If anyone had ever asked me, "what disease do you fear most?" I would have answered instantly.

"Breast cancer."

Breast cancer could happen to me. I was being asked to go behind the statistics and the scientific studies of a disease that kills thousands of women each year. I was being asked to look beyond the diagnosis to the tears and terrors of women who could be me. I was being asked to give a voice to my own fear, to give a face to breast cancer.

For Erica Berger, the colleague who would take her camera to the heart of darkness and come out with hope, the assignment was even more powerful. In 1976, her father was diagnosed with cancer. Erica had just been accepted by the University of Florida but she stayed home instead, working as a legal secretary for the last year of her father's life. She enrolled a month after he died, shaken not just by the disease but by a year of reaching out to her father and rarely connecting. From early on, the assignment would hit her with the pain of her own past.

Erica and I went forward into a place shadowed by every woman's fears. It didn't take me long to hang a card in my shower showing how to do a breast self-exam. And just a few months into the assignment, I decided that at the age of thirty-eight it was time for my first mammogram. During the year and a half we worked together, Erica underwent two sonograms to rule out a suspicious lump.

From the beginning, we knew that some of the women whose lives we were about to enter might die. That made the assignment even more difficult. These were the lives of real women who were not just breast-cancer patients but who also were mothers and daughters and wives and sisters.

First we had to find the right lives to enter. This would be a months-long process of sitting in on support groups, talking to social workers and surgeons and oncologists, interviewing almost 150 women diagnosed with breast cancer. That's how we met the brave and caring women whose stories make up this book. Women who would let us into their lives during the most traumatic times of triumph and tragedy they would ever experience.

Women like Sue Rosenbaum, a forty-two-year-old artist and gardener who was about to become a grandmother and also had a pre-school-age daughter, and whose breast cancer had already metastasized to her brain. Like Fran Lenzo, a varsity talker with a double mastectomy, whose husband was at her side every step of the way. Like Liz LoRusso, who was fighting to remain an active mother to her young son and daughter even as she fought the cancer that had spread to her hip and spine and pelvis. Like Lorraine Timmes, a medical miracle who spent seven straight years on chemotherapy and survived metastatic breast cancer. Like Cathy Langan, whose stage-three breast cancer failed to destroy her dream of having a baby. And like the Florio sisters, four very different women bound together not only by blood but by the disease that stalked their family like a serial killer.

With each of them and the ten other women whose stories we would show and tell, Erica and I couldn't be content with rapport. We had to build relationships. There had to be trust and understanding and even commitment before Fran Lenzo could describe the night she decided that if she was going to be bald, she was going to be bald on her own terms—the night she picked up her Lady Shick and handed her husband Jerry his Norelco and they shaved off the patches of coffee-brown hair that had yet to be claimed by chemotherapy. Before Fran could let Erica photograph her as she lay vulnerable on a cold metal table with her scarred chest marked for radiation. Before Sue Rosenbaum could invite us to the baby shower for her older daughter and the pizza party for her three-year-old's birthday. Before Sue could let us sit with her as doctors told her that further treatment was useless. We held each other in a hospital treatment room that day and all three of us cried.

Even for those who survive, the shadows remain. Survival does not mean that life will go back to the way it was. Breast cancer survivors mourn the past and redefine the future. They redefine themselves. For good or for bad, their lives will never be the same. If a theme dominates their stories of loss and reconstruction, it is that change is the universal outcome of a disease that scars the spirit as well as the body.

For some women, the aftermath of breast cancer means depression—questions they can't answer, anxieties they can't shake, fears they can't dispel. Survival means shock and anger and denial. And, after a while, it can mean discoveries about their own strengths and abilities and new meanings for old connections— for marriage and motherhood and love and friendship.

For a year and a half, my friend Erica Berger and I walked in other women's sunshine and shadows. What follows are stories of grief and grace and caring and courage. Stories of women and their families confronting the challenge of breast cancer.

Stories for all of us. As Erica and I learned, we're all in this together.

Irene Virag

CHAPTER ONE

"We're in This Together": Heartbreak, Hope and Laughter

For the past nine months, breast cancer has ruled the nights and days of Fran and Jerry Lenzo's marriage. Nights and days of heartbreak and hope. Nights and days of sorrow and sweetness.

Like the snow-flecked night in January five months after the day Fran first felt a lump under her right armpit. She'd already had a double mastectomy and she was just starting chemotherapy. Fran's collar-length hair had been cropped short and she'd bought two wigs. She'd told Jerry what she wanted to do.

"My hair is the one thing I have control over," she explained just after New Year's, on the morning she looked in the mirror and realized she no longer had eyebrows. "I don't want to wait for the chemo to take my hair. If I'm going to be bald I want to be bald on my terms." Still, Jerry was shaken that night by the sight of his wife standing in the hall with a clump of her coffee-brown hair in her hand. "Look at this," she said. And she yanked another handful of hair from her head. "Tell me this isn't happening."

Jerry cradled his wife in his arms. He ran his fingers through her hair as he'd done so many times before in their seven years of marriage, but now it was different. Now Jerry Lenzo watched silently as the strands of his wife's hair floated to the kitchen floor. He kissed her lashless eyelids. "You're beautiful," he whispered.

Fran and Jerry are varsity talkers. They love telling anyone who'll listen that they can drive hundreds of miles to Pennsylvania and never click on the car radio because they have so much to talk about. Dave Scheiner, Jerry's longtime buddy who spent the day in the hospital with him when Fran had surgery, jokes that the couple's friends need gadgets on their phones to say, "Yeah Lenzo, uh-huh, uh-huh," at the push of a button. "That way, he doesn't even know you went out to dinner. He just keeps talking."

But the rest of that winter evening, the talkers held their thoughts to themselves. They had a quiet dinner and later they sat in their beige recliners watching a rerun of "Cheers." When Jerry turned off the television and Fran packed away her crocheting, the silence intruded.

"It's time," Fran announced.

"I don't want to, Fran. I can't."

"Please, Jerry. You promised."

She took him by the hand to the upstairs bathroom. She had everything ready. A chair faced the mirror over the sink. A pair of barber scissors lay on the toilet seat. Two electric shavers were plugged in and waiting. Fran sat down and handed her husband the scissors.

"It's okay. I'm ready."

"I love you," he said.

He cut off her hair and then Fran picked up her Lady Schick; Jerry turned on his Norelco and they shaved away what was left. It took almost an hour. When they were finished, Jerry vacuumed the hair from the bathroom floor. He went into the bedroom and waited for his wife to emerge from the shower. He was used to the scars on her chest. Now she was also totally bald.

Fran looked in the mirror. "I look pretty good with no hair."

Jerry touched her white scalp. "It feels like number two grit sandpaper. You have a beautiful head, my little Chia Pet."

"I'm balder than you are."

"I have bigger breasts."

They cracked up laughing.

That's the way it is with Fran and Jerry Lenzo. This is their story.

A story about breast cancer.

A love story.

He was a forty-two-year-old father of two boys who was going through a divorce. She was a thirty-seven-year-old widow with a daughter and a handicapped son. They already knew each other; Fran was a secretary at an electronics firm that used the Minuteman Press franchise Jerry owned. One afternoon, Jerry phoned to ask about two groups she belonged to—a diet program and Parents Without Partners. The conversation ran on and Fran suggested that they get together for tea.

It was very suburban. They met at a diner. Not that a crowd would have inhibited them, but it was nine o'clock on a Monday night in November and they practically had the place to themselves. They ate cherry cheesecake and drank tea and by their own description they talked and talked and talked.

On their third date, they went bowling. Afterward, as they ran across the street to the car, Fran touched Jerry's arm.

"I think I love you," she said.

"I think I love you too."

They kissed. "When two people are in love," Jerry said, "they should get married."

Fran laughed. "So when do you want to get married?"

The wedding invitation they sent out soon afterward said the rest:

This day
I will marry My Friend
The One I laugh with, live for,
dream with,
Love.

On April 21, 1985, Frances Mary Teresa Franco Sensale, a welder's daughter who grew up in a New Jersey suburb she calls Leave-It-to-Beaver Land, married Gerard Peter Lenzo, a clothing salesman's son who grew up in the Bedford-Stuyvesant neighborhood of Brooklyn and always wanted to be a printer. The bride wore a pink street-length dress. The groom wore a black suit and pink tie. They hosted a reception for thirty-eight guests and danced to Anne Murray's "Nobody Loves Me Like You Do" at the restaurant where they'd had their second date.

Two people in love got married. And even breast cancer hasn't kept them from trying to live happily ever after.

They lived in a house in Huntington on Long Island's north shore—in a cedar-shingled, center-hall colonial on a dead-end street with a deck in the back and a magnolia tree in the front. Fran helped with Jerry's printing business. They went on weekend drives; they ate out a lot. Every year, they went back to Cove Haven, a resort in the Pocono Mountains of Pennsylvania where they spent their honeymoon.

They'd been married more than seven years when Fran discovered the lump. She was working out with six-pound hand-weights in the exercise room just off the master bedroom. She felt a muscle pull. She rolled up her pink T-shirt and rubbed under her armpit and along the side of her right breast. She felt something. A hard knot. As big as a golf ball. She touched it again—then she went back to her workout.

That night, she showed the lump to Jerry. They both figured it was a pulled muscle or a blind pimple, nothing to worry about. It was late August or early September 1992—Fran didn't think it was important enough to note the date. Every couple of days, she'd feel the lump but it never got bigger or harder—so she never anguished over it.

Still, when she saw an ad in the newspaper about mammograms at their local hospital, she decided to go. That wasn't until October 9—a day that is black-lettered in the calendar of Fran Lenzo's mind. The day she had her very first mammogram. She was told she had a lump in her left breast as well and three hours later, she was in a surgeon's office. Somewhere along the way, she called Jerry at work. "Something's going on," she told him.

One week later, they found out exactly what. A biopsy showed the hard knot was a malignant tumor. And there was a suspicion of cancer in her left breast. Jerry took the call from the surgeon. When he hung up, he walked over to his wife. "It's cancer," he whispered. Fran froze—and then her disbelief shook the room. "How could it be?" she screamed. "It can't be." Jerry held her as she beat her fists against his chest.

The next morning, Fran was holding Jerry's hand when the surgeon told her they wouldn't know for sure if she'd need a single or a double mastectomy until they operated.

They spent a dizzying week getting second and third opinions. "My whole life was up in the air and I felt numb," Fran said. "I wanted to be numb because I didn't want to feel—because if I felt, then I'd think and if I thought, then I'd cry and if I cried, I'd go crazy. . . . Diabetes was always my lot in life. I'm insulin-dependent. I always assumed that one day I'd die of complications from diabetes. Then, all of a sudden, it was like, my God, I'm going to die tomorrow of breast cancer. I read the obituaries every day. I'd look for women; I'd look at their ages—thirty-six, thirty-nine, forty-six, fifty-two. I'd think, she must have had breast cancer. And I'd wonder about what wasn't in the paper. Did she have a mastectomy? How much and what kind of chemo? Did she try a bone marrow transplant? How long do I have before my obituary is in the paper?"

Together Fran and Jerry read books about breast cancer. They weighed their options—and they talked. They scheduled the mastectomy for October 30.

A week before the surgery, Jerry called Fran's two younger sisters. One of them phoned Fran's daughter, Christine. If there were hard moments in the marriage, they revolved around Fran's children. Her son, Jimmy, had cerebral palsy and behavioral problems and a few months after their wedding, they had to put the eleven-year-old in a home hundreds of miles away in Pennsylvania. And Fran and Christine didn't get along.

"It blew my mind that she was getting married so soon after my father died," Christine says. "It was just a few years. I was ten when he died. He was my best friend. I was so angry at her—she was always such a talker but she never talked to me. She was preoccupied with my little brother. I was in the wedding party and I stood at the altar and burst into tears. They weren't tears of joy.

"From the beginning, I had a real attitude toward my mother and I had an even bigger attitude toward Jerry. I thought my mother was a wimp and he was a tyrant who controlled her and I got the short end of the stick every time."

Christine lasted one semester at Westchester University in Pennsylvania. "I partied all the time and my grades weren't good. My mother said she wouldn't pay for it anymore."

When Christine came home, the arguments resumed. Seven months later, Fran and Jerry told her to find another place to stay. In silence, the eighteen-year-old went to live on her own—the mother and daughter never even said good-bye.

Time only hardened the rift. Fran and Christine hadn't spoken for a year and a half when Christine answered the phone at 11:30 on a Saturday night. Just the week before she had thrown a birthday card from her mother into the trash. And now two words changed everything.

"As soon as I heard the words breast cancer, it took me about one second to decide what I was going to do," Christine says. "It was almost midnight but as soon as I stopped crying, I called her. I said, 'Mommy, let's forget everything and start over.' The next day Jerry invited me and my boyfriend to come over."

At first mother and daughter walked on eggshells. Fran showed Christine the changes in the house—the teenager's bedroom had been converted into a billiard room and her walk-in closet was cleared for a pinball machine. And in the living room Fran sat down at a new Baldwin to demonstrate the fruits of her recent piano lessons. The song she played is called "If We Hold on Together" and if that seems like something out of a soap opera, well, Fran often says, "My life's a soap opera." That day, as they embraced, a parent and child washed away years of anger with their tears.

Before Christine left, Fran brought out a copy of her mammogram. They talked about breast cancer and mastectomies. And then Fran guided Christine's hand over the right side of her breast and pressed her fingers into the hard knot she'd felt during a workout that already seemed so long ago.

"Feel this," Fran said. "This is wrong. This is what I pray you'll never feel—but if you ever do, Christine, promise me you'll go to a doctor that very same day." Then she showed her daughter how to do a breast self-exam—something Fran herself had never done.

On October 30, Christine sat all day at Huntington Hospital with Jerry and his friend Dave Scheiner and Jerry's niece. She was with Jerry when he took a call from the operating room. He didn't say a word, but his eyes were wet as he heard the doctor say that both breasts had to be removed.

Christine remembers her stepfather looked like a broken man. She rushed to comfort him. They held on to each other and Christine thought to herself: "Jerry really loves my mother. . . . Oh God, what's going to happen to my mother?"

The morning after Fran came home, her surgeon, Dr. William Martin, telephoned Jerry at work. He asked Jerry to come to his office so they could talk in person.

Jerry recalls their conversation vividly.

"There are more nodes than we like to think about," the doctor said.

Jerry was immediately alarmed. The doctor was talking about lymph nodes, chains of little bubbles that carry fluid throughout the body. The more nodes that test positive for cancer the more ominous the prognosis. Ten or more suggests that the cancer has spread significantly.

"How many?" Jerry remembers asking.

"The numbers are on the high side."

"What are you trying to tell me?"

Dr. Martin told him there had been two tumors in the right breast and one in the left. Three lymph nodes on the right tested positive for cancer; on the left eleven tested positive. Fran would need aggressive chemotherapy, possibly radiation. She was also a candidate for bone marrow transplantation—a new treatment for breast cancer. The patient's healthy bone marrow is removed and the body is bombarded with high doses of chemotherapy. Then the bone marrow is put back in the body.

It all seemed unreal to Jerry, who remembers thinking, No, please no. Everything's going too fast. A month ago we never gave breast cancer a thought. What does this mean? Is she going to die?

Two days later, when they met the oncologist, Dr. Michael S. Buchholtz, Jerry pulled him aside: "I told Fran she only had eight nodes involved."

Jerry remembers the oncologist's answer: "She has to know. She'll have to consider bone marrow transplantation. She should be making that decision soon."

Fran came back into the room and the doctor told her. "I couldn't relate to the numbers," Fran recalls. "I still can't. But I got teary-eyed—because Jerry wanted to protect me and I loved him even more for it. And because I thought, wow, we're really in this together. I can't die, we have a great love story going on here."

Four days after Christmas, Fran started chemotherapy. She and Jerry learned a new vocabulary—Zofran, Cytoxan, Adriamycin, Fluorouracil or 5-FU. The names of the drugs that are injected into the bloodstream and that kill any existing cancer cells, no matter how tiny, hiding in the body. Drugs she received through a catheter that had been inserted on the right side of her chest two weeks before.

Jerry learned to clean the plastic tubes that dangled from a small incision just above his wife's mastectomy scars—two lines that ran from under each armpit to almost the center of her chest. Two wavy lines, each about nine inches long, that were still pink and swollen and tender to the touch.

From the beginning, the catheter was uncomfortable, but Fran was more concerned about the chemo. "I'd heard horror stories," she said. She recorded her chemo schedule on the calendar—UGH! days she called them. Jerry printed up yellow signs that shouted DO IT AND GET THROUGH IT in black capitals. They hung the signs throughout the house—on the mirror of Fran's vanity, above the mantel in the den, on the refrigerator door.

She designated an old pair of blue pants and a faded long-sleeve shirt as her throw-up outfit and she wore it to almost every chemo session. She always carried a yellow plastic basin—the kind hospital patients brush their teeth in—just in case she got sick. "Getting chemo is like having a virus," Fran says, "you feel tired and achy and queasy and just not right."

Jerry always went with her. He'd massage her feet while the anti-nausea drug Zofran dripped into her body. He'd hold her hand while the nurse pushed syringes filled with Adriamycin, the drug that causes hair loss, and the other medications through the catheter tube.

For the next two months, in two-week cycles, Fran went to her oncologist's office. The first Tuesday, she'd get a one-and-a-half-hour treatment she called Big Chemo and the following Tuesday she'd get a thirty-minute Little Chemo. Then she was off for two weeks. Ten days after the treatment started, Fran lost her pubic hair. A few days later, she stood in the front hall with a clump of coffee-brown hair in her hand. And that evening, she and Jerry went upstairs and shaved her head.

In March, the chemotherapy was suspended while Fran underwent tests for the bone marrow transplant. Jerry held his wife's hand while Dr. Buchholtz extracted bone marrow samples from her hip.

"Ow, ow," Fran yelled at one point.

"It's okay. You're all right." Jerry squeezed her hand to reassure her.

"OW."

"What's wrong?" Jerry asked.

"My hand. You're holding it too tight."

Almost five months to the day after she underwent the double mastectomy, Fran felt pressure building in her chest. She couldn't lie down without choking. Jerry rushed her to the emergency room. When she went home, she was still uncomfortable. The next day she called her family physician. "When I lie down, my face gets red as a beet and swells up," she told him. "I feel like a kielbasa ready to blow up." She was readmitted. Tests showed a blood clot near the catheter. Within hours, Fran was in intensive care.

She realized how fragile her body was, how much could go wrong. Her new insurance carrier refused to pay for the bone marrow transplant, which is considered experimental. Mostly because they were afraid of the procedure to begin with, Fran and Jerry decided not to go through with it.

"Are you sure?" Jerry asked. "If there's a recurrence later on, will we say it's because you didn't do the bone marrow?"

"I'll take my chances."

They were both relieved by the decision.

By the end of the month, Fran was back in ICU with another blood clot. The catheter would have to be removed. Fran's forty-sixth birthday was two days away and Jerry was planning a party.

"Don't worry," Fran said. "I'll be there."

She was.

The party sprawled across the house and yard—almost 100 friends and relatives. Fran's sisters and her mother, Clara Franco. Jerry's sons, Gary and Steven, and his brother, Richard, from California, and his mother, Rose, who Fran says is in charge of prayers. Many of the guests hadn't seen Fran since she was diagnosed. A man in a tuxedo played the accordion and a woman in a white top hat and tails delivered a singing telegram. Jerry's present to his wife was parked in the driveway—a white Eldorado with a CD player and a sunroof that was topped with a giant red bow.

Fran wore a white silk pantsuit, gold-sequined slippers, the diamond-and-ruby ring Jerry bought her two weeks before for their eighth anniversary—and a short, coffee-brown wig. "She looks so good," one guest told Jerry, "I didn't recognize her."

"She got her hair done," he said.

"I love you all, each and every one of you," Fran told her guests as Jerry looked at her adoringly from across the kitchen, his basset-hound eyes brimming with tears. "And my husband—if there is ever a man to have in your life it's Gerard Peter Lenzo. You've brought me more love and laughter and everything you can think of that's positive and good . . ."

Jerry blew her a kiss. He walked over to her and they embraced. Everyone applauded.

"Can I take off my hair now?" she said.

Nine days after the party, Fran was back at Dr. Martin's office to have a temporary catheter inserted in her neck so she could resume chemotherapy. It was supposed to be a routine procedure with a local anesthetic.

Jerry sat in the waiting room shifting in his seat. He checked his watch—it had been almost twenty minutes. He rubbed his face. Two children sitting nearby tried to play peekaboo with him but Jerry was oblivious.

Ten minutes later, the door opened. Fran appeared in a wheelchair. Her face was as white as the hospital gown she was wearing. She held her head down and rubbed the back of her neck.

Jerry knelt in front of the wheelchair and kissed her hand.

"Jerry," she whispered.

"Fran."

"I don't know."

Jerry looked to the doctor standing in the doorway.

"We couldn't put the catheter in," Dr. Martin said. "We'll have to insert one through the groin but she'll have to go into the hospital for that."

Jerry's face dropped.

"It hurt so much," Fran told him.

They sat in the waiting room while hospital arrangements were made. Jerry wrapped his arm around his wife's shoulders. Fran leaned into his chest. She looked white and shrunken and scared. Jerry sat still and stared into the distance. His eyes were wide and frightened. A tear rolled down his cheek. He pulled her closer.

Fran was admitted to Huntington Hospital for her next two Big Chemo sessions. Dr. Martin inserted a catheter in her groin; Dr. Buchholtz pushed through the drugs. Jerry took off from work and sat by her bedside and they talked the day away.

After her last in-patient treatment, Dr. Buchholtz gave Fran the name of a radiation oncologist. "We'll see what he says. Now, let this saline solution drip and then you two put on your dancing shoes and get out of here."

With just one Little Chemo left, Fran and Jerry felt like dancing. They made a reservation to go back to the future—to Cove Haven in the Poconos. "It would be the beginning," Jerry said, "of our return to the way things used to be."

The idea of putting on a bathing suit made Fran think about a prosthesis.

In early June, she drove to a lingerie shop that carries a line of mastectomy fittings. Anne Velsor, one of the owners who measured Fran the week before, placed two gray carrying cases on the counter. Fran unzipped them and picked up one of the silicone-filled prostheses that cost $360 each.

"Is this the left or the right?" she wondered out loud. "Oooh, it feels so real." She giggled and held the breast over her blouse. "Look, there's even a nipple. I'm glad I ordered the blush color. It matches my skin."

Fran cradled the prosthesis in one hand while she felt it with the other. With the timing of a stand-up comic she paused for her punchline. "I'm feeling for lumps. Should I take them for a mammogram?"

In the dressing room, Fran examined her scars and the three scabs that formed a six-inch perpendicular line—the sites of her troublesome catheters. She put on a bra and poked the empty size 38-B cups. "It's time to fill in the blanks."

Anne Velsor showed her how to position the prostheses in specially designed bras with pockets. "I used to heave mine up and position them," Fran said. "So now I'll take them out of a box and position them. I'd rather have breasts in a box than have mine still attached and killing me."

Anne helped Fran adhere the prostheses directly to her chest using an exfoliant, a special eyebrow pencil and horseshoe-shaped adhesive and velcro strips. "I'm still numb there," Fran said. "I'll have to get used to these—like my partial plate. I just kept wearing it till I got used to it, now it's a part of me."

Fran exulted as she pulled the bra over her new breasts. "I'll go home and say, 'Feel me Jerry, feel my breasts.'

"Can I go in the hot tub with them on?"

"The jacuzzi yes, the sauna no."

Fran bounced up and down. "I can hardly wait till Jerry gets home—I'll say, 'Hi there, handsome . . .'" Fran stuck out her chest and did her best Mae West impression.

Three weeks later, she wore the prostheses to a meeting of the support group she had been attending at Huntington Hospital since she started chemotherapy.

"Notice anything different about me, girls?"

At which point, Fran yanked up her shirt. "Look, you can't tell it's not me. We went out for breakfast Saturday and I'm ordering low-fat everything and of course I'm bald as a cue ball so I tell the waitress my whole story. I say, 'Feel my new boobs, they're great, go ahead.' She did."

"May I?" a woman in a red blouse asked.

It was show-and-tell at a breast cancer support group as a prosthesis was passed from hand to hand.

"Oh my," said red blouse as she held it. "It's heavy."

"They're one pound each," Fran said. "I weighed them on my bathroom scale. I love the weight of them. With the double mastectomy, I touch myself and it's just bone there. I put the fake boobs on and I don't feel so vulnerable."

The prosthesis came full circle and Fran popped it back in her bra. "Am I balanced?" she asked.

They went to Cove Haven on the third of July and relived their honeymoon for five days. Kitsch and kissing. They drove in the white shuttle bus known as "The Love Machine." They played "The Newlywed Game" and slow-danced and strolled in the woods. They slept in a round bed and took bubble baths in a red heart-shaped tub.

At dinner the first night, Fran wore the white pantsuit she bought for her birthday party and no wig. The woman across the table asked if she was getting chemotherapy. Fran told her story.

The next morning before breakfast, she studied her husband. "You're so quiet. What's the matter?"

"Nothing."

"Tell me. You were quiet at dinner last night."

"Why'd you have to talk about it so much? All you talked about was breast cancer."

"That woman was asking me questions. What was I supposed to do, not answer her?"

"It was all so somber. Listening to you, all I could think was I don't want the five days to be like this. We need a break from breast cancer, Fran."

"Talking about it is my way of dealing with it, Jerry. I have to be me."

"I love you the way you are. But you should've seen their faces. And then when you said you're diabetic, they all looked like, 'My God, is this woman going to make it through dinner?'"

The next night Fran wore a coffee-brown wig. Her head was sweating and she whispered to Jerry that she was going to the restroom to take off her hair.

"I'll help you," Jerry said. He reached up and in one swoop he pulled off her wig.

"Thank you," Fran said. Everyone laughed.

Breast cancer still stalks the nights and days of Fran and Jerry Lenzo's marriage.

"Fran Lenzo falls into a very undesirable statistical category," Dr. Buchholtz says. "Statistically, fifty-five to eighty-five percent of breast cancer patients with ten nodes involved will relapse within five years and eighty percent will relapse within three years. . . . Nobody knows on an individual level what's going to happen. Chemotherapy is insurance. Chemotherapy will lower the probability of recurrence. If in five years she doesn't have a recurrence, then the chemotherapy was effective. If her cancer never comes back, then the chemo was very effective. Short of waiting to see what happens, you really can't tell.

"Everyone deals with it in their own way. The thing that amazes me—no matter how they do it, most people come to grips with it and do what they have to do. People find a courage and capacity to rise up to this disease. I must say though, Fran's more upbeat than most. Fran Lenzo has a wonderful sense of humor."

A few days after they returned from Cove Haven, Fran went on tamoxifen and started a six-week course of radiation. The map of radiation fields had already been drawn on her chest—dots and lines, circles and Xs in indelible ink. Now, Fran visits the office of Dr. Richard Byrnes, where she lies on a computer-operated linear accelerator inside a five-feet-thick concrete vault and gets zapped with a dosage of radiation strong enough to annihilate any microscopic cancer cells still lurking inside her.

Alone in the room, Fran reassures herself with meditation. She has a simple mantra—the words "good health."

The daily treatments will go on until August 20, when Fran plans to take her husband to Atlantic City for his fifty-first birthday. After that, she'll visit her oncologist for check-ups every two months and hope for a happy ending.

Fran and Jerry hope in tandem. They light up the dark corners with tenderness. They turn the unspeakable into one-liners. They scatter the shadows with laughter.

A week ago, they sat in their beige recliners and talked. It was like the heart-to-hearts that had taken on a new dimension when breast cancer entered their nights and days. Conversations they call "phillies" or philosophicals.

"Do you remember when we first got married, how I'd worry that you only loved me for my breasts," Fran started. "I'd ask you, 'How would you feel if I didn't have them anymore?'"

"And I'd say, 'Don't even think like that.' I loved your breasts—Big One and Little One."

Fran laughed. "Yeah. One was a size C, the other was a B. And you'd ask me, 'Has anyone ever told you you have beautiful breasts?' In those days, Jerry, you were an all-American breast man."

"Breasts seem almost frivolous now," Jerry said. "Having a wife who is your best friend, that's what's important in a marriage."

Fran looked at her husband. "You never cringed, you never made me feel like less of a woman. I never felt spurned."

"I still think you're sexy."

"Sometimes it makes me want to cry when you say that, but I always choose to believe you."

"Fran, I wasn't joking when I told you, the doctor can keep your breasts as long as I get the rest. We're in this together. I'm just so happy you're alive and I can still talk to you and hold you."

Fran headed into the kitchen for lemonade. Jerry grabbed her leg as she walked by. "Anytime she passes me," he said, "she still has to watch where my hands go."

Fran laughed. "Yeah. He likes bald women."

That's how it is with Fran and Jerry Lenzo.

———

CHAPTER 2

Lorraine Timmes: A Survivor

Lorraine Timmes remembers looking out her hospital window at a bleak concrete courtyard before her mastectomy and thinking her life was over. She remembers her sixteen-year-old twin daughters coming to visit and how her ten-year-old son stood in the courtyard and waved to her because he was too young to be allowed into her room. She remembers praying to God to please let her live long enough to see her boy grow up.

Her son, David, is a thirty-three-year-old project engineer for a communications company now. And Lorraine Timmes is something of a medical miracle. Her oncologist says she may not be one in a million, but she is at the very least one in a thousand.

Lorraine Timmes is a survivor of metastatic breast cancer. She survived cancer that spread to her bones—to her spine and even to her skull. A widespread metastasis that put her chances of survival at eighteen percent.

The chronology of her ascent from hell blazes in her memory—the signposts like tapers in a dark cave. She was in the shower when she first felt the pea-sized lump on the outside of her right breast. It was a January night in 1972. She was thirty-nine years old, legally separated from her husband and living with their children in a split-level in the mid-Island community of Bethpage. She called her gynecologist the next morning, but he didn't even have her come in for a checkup. So she called her family doctor, who examined her and said it was nothing to worry about. She waited another three weeks then went to a friend's gynecologist. He sent her for a mammogram.

This was almost twenty-two years ago when cancer was something to be ashamed of—when the treatment was kept almost as secret as the disease. "I had to ask what a mammogram was," Lorraine says. "I'd never even heard the word before. I'd never heard the word mastectomy either—until it was being applied to me. I didn't know a soul who'd had breast cancer."

That first mammogram didn't show anything suspicious, and the gynecologist reassured her that the pea-sized lump was probably nothing—still he suggested it be removed. The day of the surgery Lorraine was asked to sign a form giving the doctor permission to remove her breast if the lump was cancerous.

"In those days, you handed your life over to a doctor, no questions asked. But to me this was a horrendous thought. I said 'absolutely not.'"

When the doctor came into the recovery room after the biopsy that Friday night, the patient asked, "I'm all right, aren't I?"

The conversation may have happened more than two decades ago but as Lorraine observes, "These things are seared into my memory."

The doctor said, "Why don't we talk about it Monday?"

Lorraine pushed for an answer. "What's to talk about? I'm a big girl. Tell me."

A few days later Lorraine Timmes underwent a radical mastectomy.

Several weeks later when she was told her lymph nodes were clean, she decided she'd been through the worst. "I was going to tough it out. I was going to survive."

She needed armor for her psyche. She needed it to ward off the look of horror on her mother's face the first time she saw the vertical gash that ran from above her daughter's armpit to her waist. She needed it to quell the fear of recurrence that is common among breast cancer patients—a fear for which there is good reason. According to statistics, sixty percent of the recurrences appear within the first three years, twenty percent within the next two years and twenty percent in later years. And Lorraine needed it the day six weeks after surgery when she returned to her job as a legal secretary for a housing developer.

"My boss was fired while I was out. I went back to a monstrous man. He said, 'I understand you've been ill. I'm glad you're back. I take my coffee with milk and sugar.' I was supposed to be back part-time, but he didn't give me a break. I'd sit and sob into my typewriter—we used manual typewriters in those days and let me tell you after a radical mastectomy it wasn't easy. But I needed my job. I remember people just didn't know what to say to me. One day I was in the model kitchen where we made coffee and one of the men came in and said, 'So what are you gonna do now, grow another one?' I looked at him and said, 'No, I don't think so.' He wrote me a note of apology later but at that moment I felt like crying."

About one year after the mastectomy, Lorraine began dating. "Breast cancer weeds the men from the boys. I didn't tell anyone until I thought they had a reason to know. Then I'd simply say, 'There's something I think you should know.' I'd tell him about the mastectomy and I'd ask, 'Would that bother you?' I had a relationship for three years and it was never a problem."

In January of 1977, Lorraine noticed an ache in her chest. She thought it was a pulled muscle. When the pain got worse, she wondered if she'd broken a rib. It never entered her mind that the pain might signal a recurrence, but she thought it could be connected to her scar. A bone scan provided no answers. She trekked to doctor after doctor—gynecologists and rheumatologists and neurologists and internists. The pain got so bad she couldn't breathe. She was put on pain killers. By now it was springtime, and Lorraine was working as a secretary in Manhattan. "I'd take codeine in the morning to get to work. I was convinced I was crazy. I went into therapy."

Finally she saw an internist who ran a battery of tests. All hell had broken loose in her body.

The cancer had traveled to her bones—the most common path of metastasis in breast cancer, accounting for almost fifty percent of recurrences. To her ribs and her sternum, to her spine and her skull. The doctor suggested her ovaries be removed to cut off the supply of estrogen to the tumors—a standard procedure in treating pre-menopausal patients at that time. She had the surgery in November and two months later she went on chemotherapy.

As bad as she thought the mastectomy was, this was worse.

"I became preoccupied with thoughts of death, my death. One night I invited my three closest women friends over. I showed them the dress I wanted to be buried in. It was a long lemon yellow dress, knit like a tube, with a little jacket. I'd worn it several times and I loved it. I knew I'd be a fabulous looking corpse. I laid it out on my bed, with the arms crossed, like it was waiting for me. I even planned the music for my funeral—a movement from Beethoven's Fifth Piano Concerto called the Emperor Concerto, which is very triumphant."

After a few chemotherapy sessions, Lorraine went on long-term disability. "I got sick right away from the chemo. There was no such thing as anti-nausea drugs like today. Once I quit working, it got easier because I could rest." By this time, her daughters, Nancy and Jeanne, were in college and she was divorced and living in the split-level with her son.

She lost her hair. "It was Farrah Fawcett's heyday and hair was in. I'd dream about hair. I never had great hair but it was hair and it was on my head. When I went for my first wig, I tried on a blond one to be funny. My hair was dark. The saleswoman said 'you have a blond face.' I agreed. So when my hair finally grew back, I stayed a blonde."

But that wouldn't be for seven long years. Seven years of chemo and baldness and pain and hanging on to hope as if it were a thin rope suspended over a sharp precipice.

She endured the pain of mouth ulcers—sometimes four or more open sores on her tongue and gums at the same time. She lived on oatmeal and milk. The chemo drugs made her bloated. She reached a point where the lemon yellow dress with the little jacket didn't fit anymore. As the months passed, her preoccupation with death disappeared. "I had my moments, but I got used to it. I was in therapy. I went out and saw friends. I'm a reader. I listened to classical music. I kept busy. I was never bored."

If she held off the enemy by day, it besieged her in darkness. One night Lorraine dreamt she'd been wrapped in a blanket and dropped down a deep pit. She was struggling to free herself but kept getting more tangled in the blanket. The more she struggled, the faster she fell. She hit the bottom of the pit. She awoke from her dream, knowing she'd died. She couldn't go back to sleep.

"I was at my lowest at that time—it was about halfway through the chemo. Maybe I was dying. I had neuropathy, when the chemo interferes with your nerves. My mouth was pulled up on one side like I'd had a stroke."

And then, after she had been on chemo for six years, her doctors thought the cancer in Lorraine's body had been killed. "It was a gut feeling," says her oncologist, Dr. Larry Bilsky. "You can't rely on having one hundred Lorraine

Timmeses in a study to guide you. Somehow something tells you to stop." During the next year, the dosage was decreased gradually and the intervals between sessions got longer. Her oncologist made a champagne toast at her last chemo session. Lorraine remembers her response: "I hope I never see you again."

About six months later, she looked in her bathroom mirror and a pair of bright eyes stared back at her. The olive green pallor had gone from her face and her color was good. Lorraine Timmes looked at herself and smiled.

Since then, Lorraine, who is now sixty-one and lives in an apartment, has gone to work as an executive secretary for a department store. She went back to her oncologist once or twice after the champagne toast, but "I'd get shaky and sick in the lobby. I stopped going in 1984. My internist takes care of me now."

"When we decided to stop chemotherapy, Lorraine was very anxious," says the internist, Dr. Robert Z. Goldstein. "Chemo had become her security blanket. But she just continued to do well. I'd say Lorraine Timmes is cured—of course I use that word cautiously . . ."

The doctor gives credit to the patient. "She's a survivor—she's been through a lot, and she just kept fighting back. She's an extraordinary lady. I'd say she's lucky, and, yes, I'd assume she's an unusual patient."

Life after cancer has included two breast biopsies that frightened Lorraine but proved benign. Four years ago, her son got married. This time she didn't wear a wig as she had done at her daughters' weddings years before. Her twins are thirty-nine—the same age Lorraine was when she was diagnosed. Nancy is an editor for March of Dimes; Jeanne is a manager for an international electronics company and the mother of six-year-old Nicholas. "I worry about them. They have their checkups and their mammograms, but they're not neurotic about it. And I try not to be."

Still, the scars of the past run deep. Lorraine Timmes can't bring herself to perform self-exams. "It's too difficult emotionally. I just can't. I see my internist a couple of times a year and my gynecologist. I have two doctors checking my one breast."

But last year, for the first time, the woman who survived metastatic breast cancer didn't meet her deductible for medical expenses. And her only medical complaint was a sinus infection. The year before that she suffered back pain. But as her internist observes: "Just because Lorraine has had metastatic breast cancer doesn't mean she can't have sciatica or osteoporosis or a bulging disc—it doesn't mean she can't have normal aches and pains and be treated like just any other ordinary patient."

LORRAINE TIMMES: I was married seventeen years and I don't really remember being married. But I remember every minute of breast cancer. I remember the emotional ups and downs and being so full of despair. Once you live through something like that, everything else seems very small. I've become impatient and intolerant of ignorance and stupidity. When I know something is wrong, I want action. And I'm not afraid of dying anymore. Once you've been so close, you realize it's not the worst thing in the world. To me, living in pain and fear is more awful than death. I've already experienced unbearable and unending pain that just got worse. I know I won't die of breast cancer—I'm truly convinced that I'm cured.

I don't take anything for granted, though. I don't neglect my health. I don't really live any differently except I carry the rosary with me and I pray every day. But I'm happier these last few years than I ever was—despite the fact that I don't like getting older.

———

Edith Kmetz: A Survivor

Two days before Valentine's Day of 1990, Andy Kmetz sat in his wheel-chair at the kitchen table, paying bills. "I remember thinking, 'Hey we're doing okay,'" he recalls. "Then I heard Edith scream." The scream came from the bathroom where his wife had just done a breast self-exam before stepping into the shower. She felt a lump the size of an almond.

Edith Kmetz has an even more vivid memory of the discovery, the scream and the fear that followed—the fear that seemed unstoppable a few days later when she was diagnosed with breast cancer.

It wasn't just fear for her own life. Edith Kmetz also had to worry about her husband's. Andy is a quadriplegic and Edith is his sole caregiver. It's been that way through the eleven years of their marriage. "It takes ten people to do my job and they don't do it well," says Edith, who has to lift and wash and dress her husband. If anything happened to her, she worried, who would take care of Andy?

For both of them it was a familiar challenge. Both Edith and Andy have experience picking up the pieces of shattered lives.

When they were kids, Andy Kmetz used to ride Edith Arran around their neighborhood on the handlebars of his green Schwinn. They used to eat hot dogs at the town beach pavilion and dance to Elvis Presley records. They were in grade school when they had their first date—Andy's dad drove them to see Anthony Quinn and Sophia Loren in the movie *Attila*. By high school, Edith and Andy weren't sweethearts anymore, but they still found time to eat lunch together now and then.

They lost contact after they graduated from high school in 1964. The year Andy got his degree from Rutgers, Edith got married and settled into suburban life. Andy, who had taken ROTC in college, settled into Army life and was stationed in Germany. One night just before Christmas of 1969, the twenty-three-year-old lieutenant swerved his brand new Alfa Romeo to avoid a head-on collision on a winding mountain road. He hit a tree and was thrown from the car. His neck was broken. Andy Kmetz would have use of his right hand and arm, but not his left. He'd be able to write and with difficulty he could maneuver his wheelchair. But he couldn't move his bowels or dress himself or put himself to bed.

The twists and turns of Edith's life were unpredictably cruel as well. She was a suburban homemaker with a little girl named Thea but before her daughter's third birthday, Edith's husband was killed in a car accident. Edith was twenty-six years old—she'd been married only five years.

The young widow and the wheelchair-bound vet who had once carved their initials in a tree met again at their fifteenth high school reunion in the spring of 1979. "I saw who he was, who he is," Edith says, "I never saw the chair." Andy saw the girl he once presented with a cigar-wrapper ring but he was afraid to even dare let himself see anything more. He was afraid to hope. "I was resigned that no one would ever look at me romantically," Andy says. "I'd been out with a few women. They got dinner and drinks, I was lucky if I got a goodnight kiss. When I met Edith again, I had no visions of anything happening. I was surprised and scared when she called me."

They were married in August of 1983 in the ranch-style house they'd had built on Great Neck Creek in the south shore community of Copiague, where they had played together as children. It was a house where all the doorways are thirty-six inches wide and the bathrooms have a five-foot turning radius to accommodate a wheelchair. Where all the light switches have been lowered and the electrical outlets have been raised. And where love and laughter flourished.

Then Edith touched herself before taking a shower and life would never be the same. "It's the shock of it—you scratch an itch, rub your arm, touch your breast and in a split second you go from being a healthy person to being a cancer patient." She had a mastectomy on March 9, 1990—the seventeenth anniversary of her first husband's death. She was in the hospital for five days.

Edith's cancer left a gap in Andy's life. His sister's husband got him up in the morning and Edith's brother put him to bed. A friend slept over so he wasn't alone at night. Thea came home from college for a few days. The VA sent a nurse twice a week to provide bowel care. And each day someone drove Andy to the hospital to visit his wife.

"By the time I was released from the hospital, I wanted everyone out of my house," says Edith. "I needed to get back to our routine and hang on to what was normal."

That night Edith lifted her five-foot-nine, 193-pound husband from his wheelchair to their bed. "It's a matter of leverage," she says, "not lifting. Besides he can stand and pivot. Every once in awhile, all of a sudden he becomes a dead weight. I've never dropped him though. I accidentally dumped him out of his wheelchair on our honeymoon but that's another story.

"My doctor knew the situation. The only thing he told me I couldn't do was vacuum."

The next morning, Edith spent an hour in the shower crying for herself. "But crying didn't bring back my breast. So I got in the car and I drove to a corset shop and bought a prosthesis." And then she took care of her husband.

"I depend on Edith for daily care," Andy says. "When she's not up to it I notice. Once I'm in bed, I'm stuck. Even if she's in another room, I know she's there. It was very lonely when she was in the hospital. I was mad because she was sick and it was taking away from my life. I missed her being there for me. My attitude was, okay you lost a breast. It's not like a leg or like you're totally paralyzed. Look what I look like—all bent up like an old man. I'd say, 'Come on, hon, it's just a breast, who's gonna see, who's gonna know? So you have a scar. Put a blouse on and don't worry about it.'

"I was upset about Edith, but I also looked at it as what's going to happen to me? I know I can't survive alone. I can't even dress myself. My thoughts ran wild—How will I get up in the morning? Will I have to sell the house and go live in a VA home?

"It took me awhile to gain some insight . . . I figured, you have the operation and boom you're better. For me, . . . as time went by, things always got easier. With Edith, they got worse. She was always worried about the cancer coming back. And when she started chemo it was like a rollercoaster ride."

Edith was on a six-month regimen of chemotherapy delivered on a two-week-on, two-week-off schedule. It was like two weeks of night and two weeks of day.

Once a week during the two weeks she was on she'd go to her doctor's office for intravenously administered chemo drugs and every day she'd take other drugs in pill form. "I'd drag myself up out of bed because I had to get Andy up and dressed," Edith says. "But then I'd flop right back down."

"For two weeks out of each month, life wasn't normal," says Andy, who supports himself and his wife on his military pension and disability payments. "The next two weeks it was like nothing was wrong."

Now life has taken on new dimensions for the two forty-seven-year-olds. When Edith got sick, Andy bought a motorized scooter that attaches to his wheelchair so he could maneuver around the house more easily and do errands like go to the bank and the store. "Breast cancer gave both of us a lot more independence," he says.

"You have to choose life," says Edith Kmetz, who not only cares for her husband but works as a volunteer for Reach-to-Recovery, making hospital visits to women who've been newly diagnosed with breast cancer, and fitting wigs and prostheses for chemotherapy patients who don't have insurance. "It's very hard to be scared all the time. At some point, you either get on with your life or put your head in the oven. It's as simple and as complicated as that. There is life after breast cancer. You just have to establish a new definition of normal."

That doesn't mean Edith Kmetz is Pollyanna. "I don't know about Andy but I'd trade my new-found independence in a nanosecond if I could go back and have that thing be benign . . . I don't agree with people who say adversity makes you stronger. I'm sorry but that's a large pile of horseshit. I'm not a better person because I've had breast cancer. I was just as nice and just as good and decent before it. When I got breast cancer I thought, what did I do to deserve this?

"You know, it's a lot like losing someone you loved. In the beginning it's the first and only thing you can think about. But as time passes your every moment isn't haunted by it. Still, every time I see a V-neck dress I can't wear, every time I take a shower, every time I go to the doctor for a checkup, I remember that for the whole rest of my life I'm living with the Sword of Damocles hanging over my head."

> *EDITH KMETZ: It's hard to be scared all the time. With every ache and pain I used to think, it's back, my cancer is back. My sister-in-law who held my hand every step of the way cured me of that. One day I had a pain in my toe. I was going on and on, wringing my hands, crying, "Oh my God, oh my God, they must have missed something on my last bone scan. Did they look at my foot? Oh God, I must have forgotten to take off my shoes." My sister-in-law looked me right in the eye and said, "Oh no Edith, you must have the dreaded cancer of the big toe." It stopped me right in my tracks. Now, when my thoughts get out of control, I tell myself, "Edith your toe hurts because you stubbed it; you don't have cancer of the big toe."*

Cathy Langan: A Survivor

The white room with the pale gray carpet and walk-in closet is empty except for a wooden rocking chair and a rattan chest surrounded by two teddy bears, a little brown dog that barks and flips over when you wind it up, a white rabbit with floppy ears and a fish with orange and green stripes. At least once a day Cathy Langan slips into the room she refuses to call anything but the baby's room and sits in the wooden rocker. She cradles one of the teddy bears and dreams.

She dreams of the ruffled curtains she'll make and how the oak tree in the corner of the front yard will filter the afternoon sun as it streams through the windows. In her dreams, the room is furnished with a wooden crib and a white bassinet and she's cuddling a pink-cheeked baby in the blue-and-white sleeper that her sister was throwing away until Cathy rescued it from the trash and brought it home to keep in the walk-in closet. For as long as she can remember, Cathy Langan has dreamed of having a baby.

Nothing, not even breast cancer, has killed that dream.

The dream seemed close seven years ago when Cathy Anderson moved in with her boyfriend Tom Langan—they'd marry, have a child, buy a house. "Having a baby was always Cathy's one burning desire," Tom says.

Cathy wasn't overly concerned even when she felt a lump the size of a golf ball in her right breast three and a half years ago. Doctors who examined her didn't think she had anything to fear but recommended she have a biopsy to make sure. It never occurred to Cathy that her dream was in danger.

"I went into surgery thinking it was just a big lumpy cyst," Cathy says. "They had me sign a consent form for a mastectomy just in case. It's like when you read the list of side effects on birth control pills warning you that something like one in 10 million women will have a seizure or stroke. But you don't know anyone it's happened to and it never enters your head that you might be the one. A mastectomy seemed such a remote possibility—even the doctors told me, 'Don't worry, you're too young to have breast cancer.'"

Cathy woke up from the surgery with a tight stocking-like bandage around her chest. "No one in the recovery room talked to me, there was no eye contact even. When they wheeled me into a private room I knew. I was crying before Tom could say the words."

The lump was a three-centimeter malignant tumor and the cancer had spread to one lymph node. Just before Thanksgiving of 1990, Cathy Langan, a thirty-four-year-old drug and alcoholism counselor, was diagnosed with stage-three breast cancer. By the new year she was bald from chemotherapy. She joined a support group that she still attends but in other ways she looked away from what had happened. She bought a $150 wig, then refused to put it on. She tore it to pieces and wore turbans instead. She ate pizza and hot dogs. She smoked a pack of cigarettes a day and ate a bowl of ice cream every night.

"For months I was in shock and denial. I didn't want my life to change so I tried to pretend nothing was different. I tried to hold on to the things that gave me comfort but after awhile I couldn't pretend anymore. Then I exploded and raged with anger. When you're a cueball-head it's hard to believe you'll ever be the same person you were before."

But she held on to the constant that had always been her life raft. Sometimes in her longings, a baby cooed. If she could cradle an infant in her dreams, Cathy Langan thought, then she could quell fear in the real world.

It never occurred to Cathy that hers might be an impossible dream—not until the day in her oncologist's office when she made a joke about getting pregnant. Cathy, who was receiving chemotherapy at the time, remembers the look of surprise on the doctor's face. She remembers the doctor's "No way."

"Well, not while I'm on chemo," Cathy said. "I'm not that crazy."

The doctor put her off. "We'll talk a year after you finish chemotherapy."

When her treatment ended on May 13, 1991, Cathy marked the one-year anniversary on a calendar. And she started making changes in her life. In September, she and Tom sneaked off to Town Hall and got married. It was a warm, early fall day and she wore a prosthesis and a one-piece bathing suit under a pink dress. After the wedding, the newlyweds went to Jones Beach for a swim in the ocean.

Cathy decided not to return to work as a counselor and started a house-cleaning business instead. She gave up cigarettes and red meat—eventually she became a total vegetarian. She began working out at a gym and meditating. She prayed the rosary every day and went to healing masses. She and Tom, who now sells fax machines for Xerox, moved into a studio apartment to save money for a house—one with a spare room they could turn into a nursery.

And exactly one year to the day her chemotherapy ended, Cathy looked at the red circle on her calendar and walked into her oncologist's office.

"I was like a kid, I was so excited," she remembers.

"You know what day this is," she told the doctor. "It's my anniversary. I'm off chemo exactly one year."

Cathy recalls the doctor's response. "That's great. You're doing great."

"Great. So it's time to have a baby. I can get pregnant now, right?"

Her oncologist, Dr. Aruna Gupta, told her to wait another two years, until November 1993, to consider the possibility. The doctor said that about fifteen percent of all women who get breast cancer are in their child-bearing years, and in the past it was believed that pregnancy increased the likelihood of the spread and recurrence of the disease. But current studies show that the survival rate is the same for premenopausal breast cancer patients who get pregnant and those who don't. "No one has the answer," Gupta said. "No one really knows."

"Most doctors recommend postponing pregnancy for two to five years after treatment. As far as I'm concerned, I told her she should wait up to three years," Gupta says today. "Of course, now she's close to forty and that becomes a whole other issue not related to breast cancer."

In the meantime, there were complications. Shortly after the one-year anniversary, a Pap test showed a pre-cancerous condition of the cervix. Since then, she's undergone a biopsy and has a Pap test every three months. And although there has been no recurrence of the breast cancer, a lump developed recently just below the mastectomy scar that turned out to be benign.

Cathy's gynecologist offers some hope. According to the gynecologist, three consecutive Pap tests have to be normal before Cathy can try to get pregnant.

And no matter what, Cathy Langan, a cancer survivor for three-and-a-half years, continues to dream her dream. "The idea of having a baby has been the light at the end of the tunnel. I would have given up a long time ago if I didn't have this dream to hang on to. I've wanted a baby so bad for so long. Ten years ago if anyone would've told me you'll marry a man who loves you madly even though you have only one breast, I'd have laughed and said, 'no way, never, they don't exist.' So I've learned to never say never."

And she won't. If the doctors persuade Cathy not to get pregnant, then she and Tom will try to adopt a child.

In January, they bought a house—a two-story contemporary in Amityville with wood floors and a fireplace and a view from the master bedroom of the Great South Bay in the distance. And a white room with pale gray carpet and a walk-in closet, where Cathy Langan can sit in a rocking chair and cradle a teddy bear. Where Cathy Langan can dream.

CATHY LANGAN: When you look good and you've re-entered life again, you start to feel alone out there because everyone's forgotten what you've been through. The people around you can afford that kind of denial—you can't. I have to look at myself every morning, I have to put on a prosthesis. When I go into a dressing room and I see there are no curtains on the stalls I think, "well, I didn't really want to try that blouse on." Even in my dreams, my oncologist always seems to be lurking in a corner somewhere. I try so hard but I can't seem to close the door on it. If you've had breast cancer you'll always have an issue to deal with. That's why I still go to a support group. I believe my emotional health is more important to my physical well-being than anything else. I don't keep things bottled up. I meditate, I do visualization and guided imagery to chase away cancer cells. I sit in the sauna at the health club and talk to my immune system. I don't eat meat or fish. I do all the things I thought only kooks do. I'd sit in a hut with a witch doctor if it kept my cancer away. I've looked at death down the barrel of a chemo tube. I'll never be the same again.

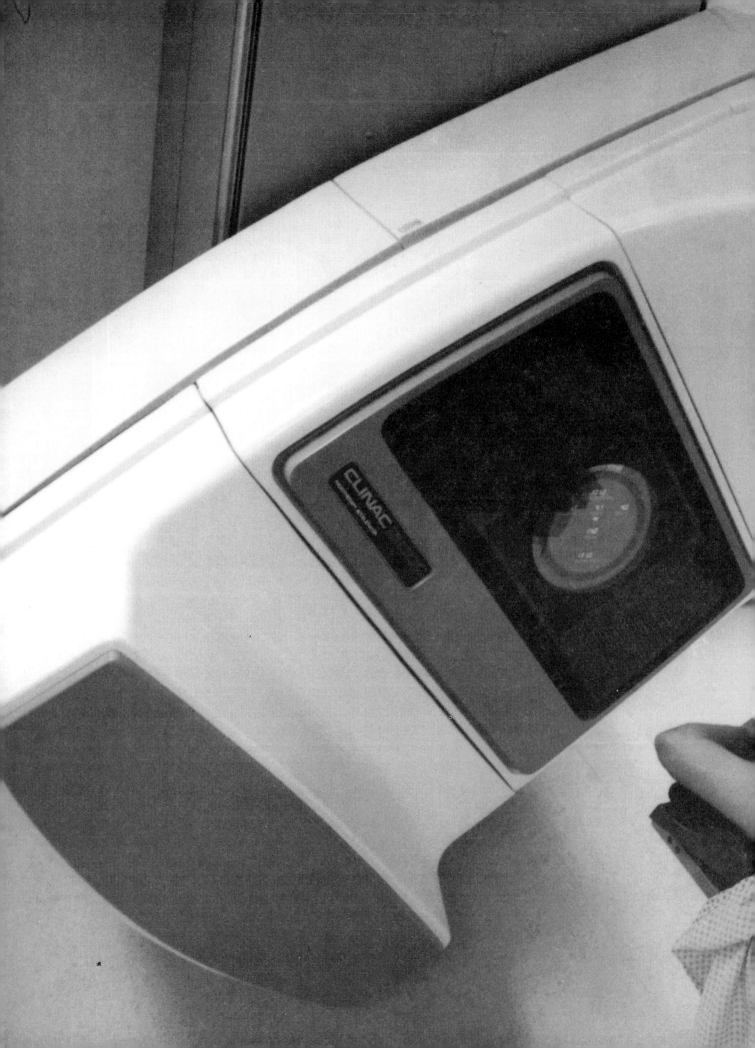

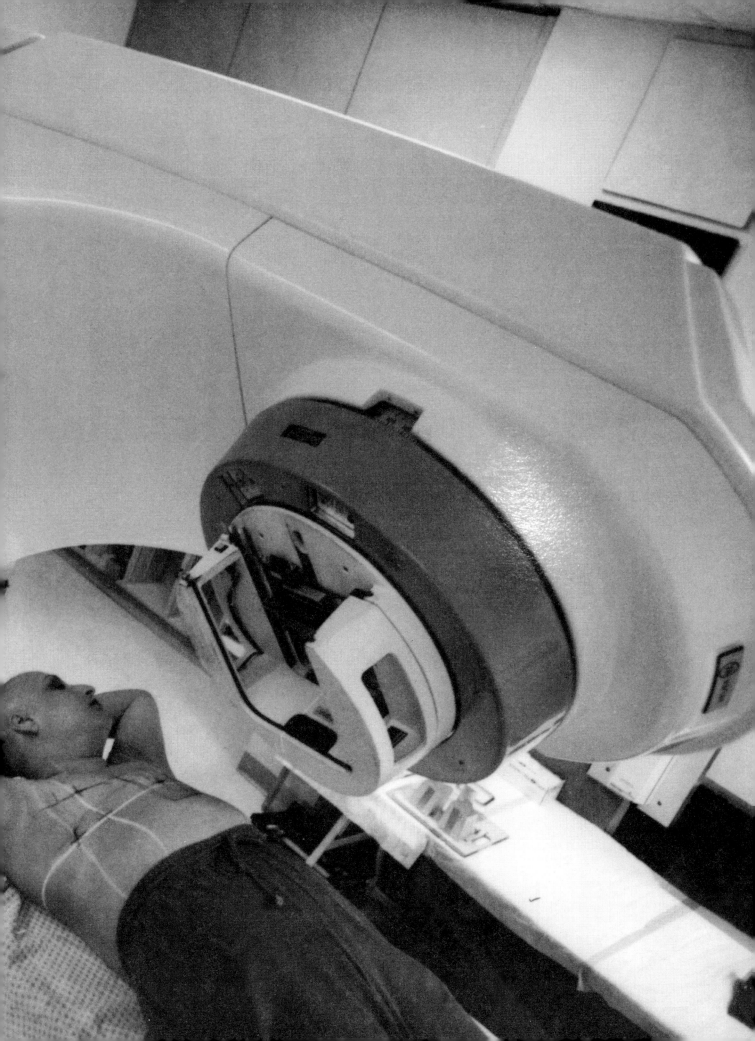

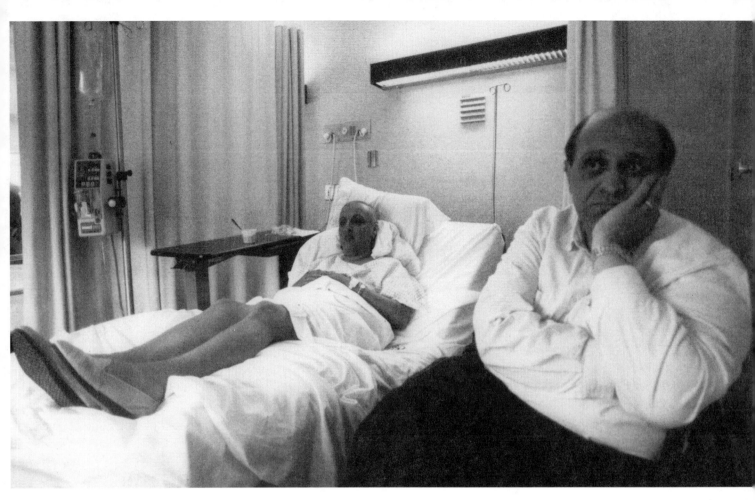

Do it and get through it
While last "Big Chemo" treatment flows into Fran Lenzo's bloodstream, her husband, Jerry, can only wait.

A time to be silent
Inside a five-foot-thick concrete vault, with the map
of radiation fields drawn on her chest in indelible
ink, Fran completes a six-week course of therapy.

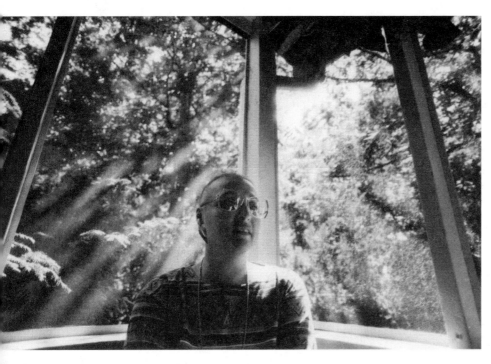

A time to speak
A few days after the last chemo treatment,
Fran turns the unspeakable into one-liners,
scattering the shadows with laughter.

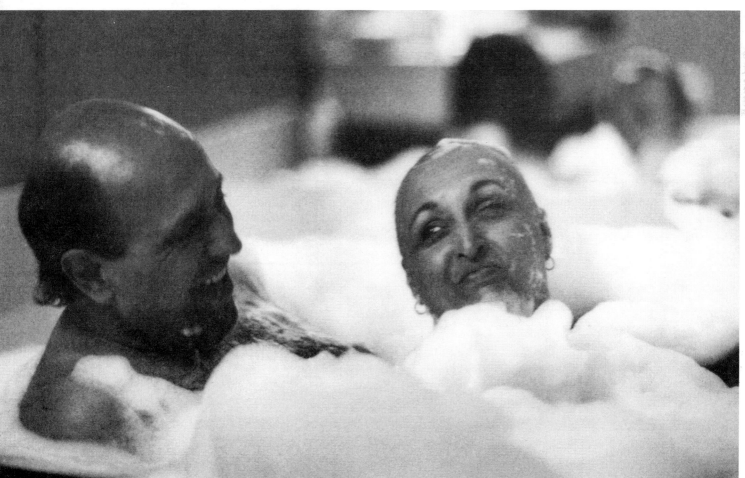

Hope in tandem
In the heart-shaped bathtub of their annual second-honeymoon hideaway, Fran and Jerry make reservations for the future. Together, like they do everything. "I'm just so happy you're alive," Jerry tells her later, "and I can still talk to you and hold you."

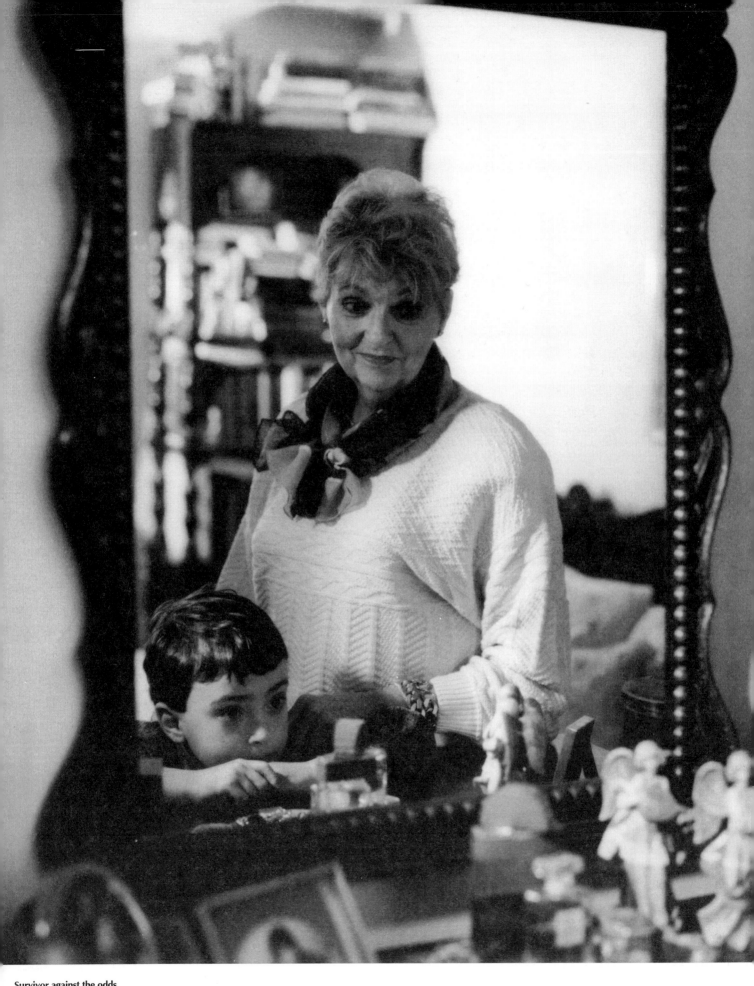

Survivor against the odds
Though her cancer had spread to her spine and skull, Lorraine Timmes is a survivor. Here with her 6-year-old grandson, Nicholas, she says, "I'd never heard the word 'mastectomy' . . . until it was being applied to me. I didn't know a soul who'd had breast cancer."

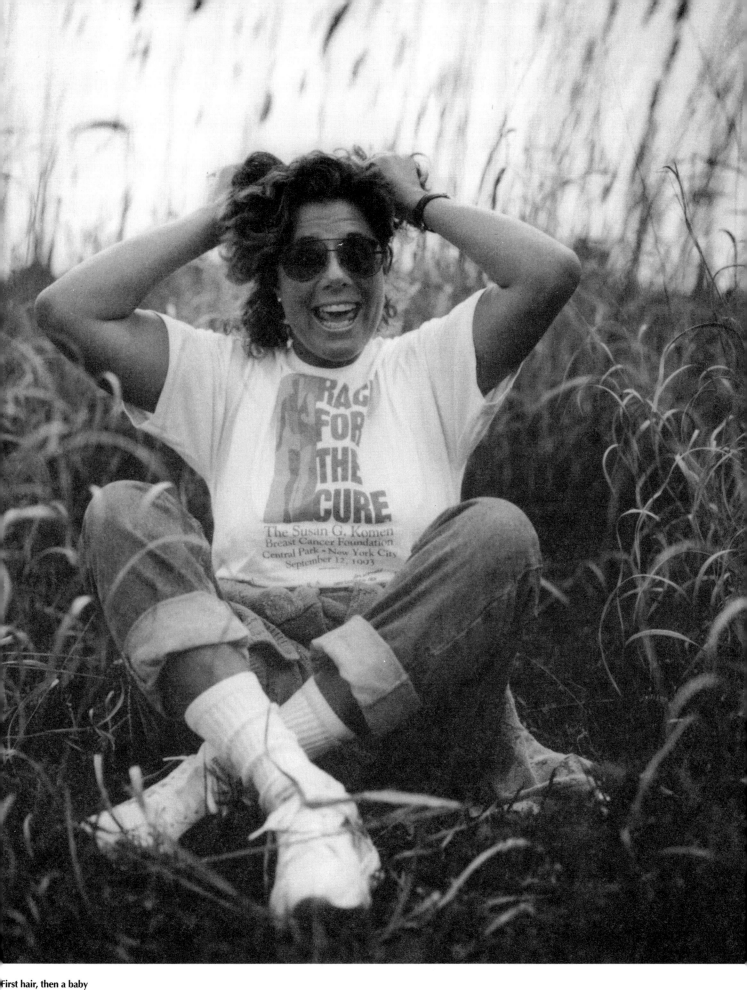

First hair, then a baby
For as long as she can remember, Cathy Langan dreamed of having a baby. At 38, she is four years cancer-free and waiting for the medical OK. "Ten years ago, if anyone would've told me you'll marry a man who loves you madly even though you have only one breast, I'd have laughed and said, 'No way, never, they don't exist.' So I've learned to never say never."

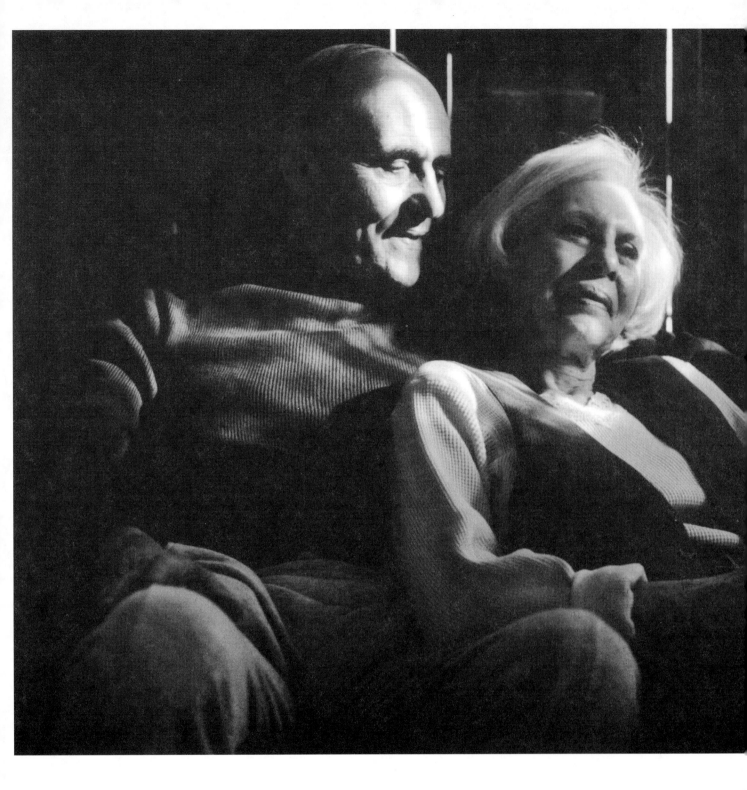

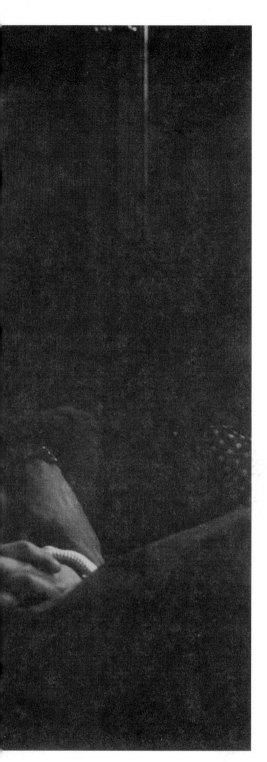

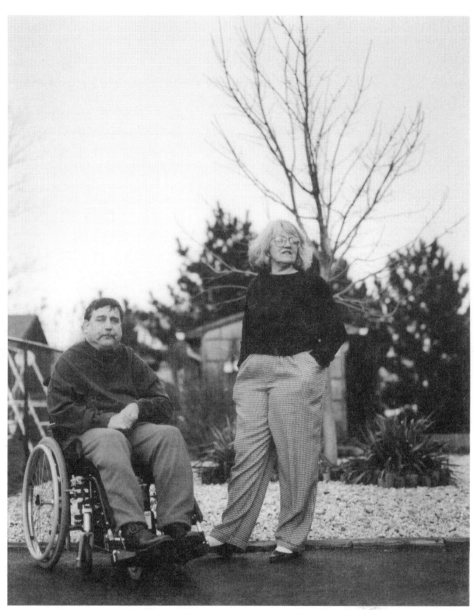

the artist's eye

elen Meyrowitz, with husband Sid, needed a year following
rgery before she could deal with the idea that she had lost
mething. "The breast is such a goddamn symbol. . . .After
while you have to let yourself mourn your loss in order to
ove on."

Keeping life in control

When she came home from the hospital
after her mastectomy, Edith Kmetz lifted
her paralyzed 5-foot-9, 193-pound
husband from his wheelchair into bed. "I
wanted—and I needed—to get back to our
routine and hang onto what was normal."

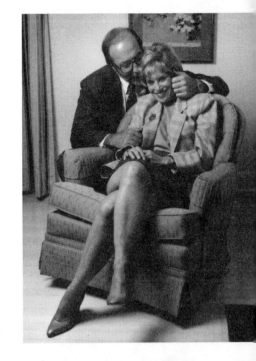

You're my everything
Cindy Bluming had an immediate reconstruction after her mastectomy. "I wanted to wake up as close to normal as possible." Her husband, Sid, says, "For both of us breast cancer was a life-altering event and we can't go back."

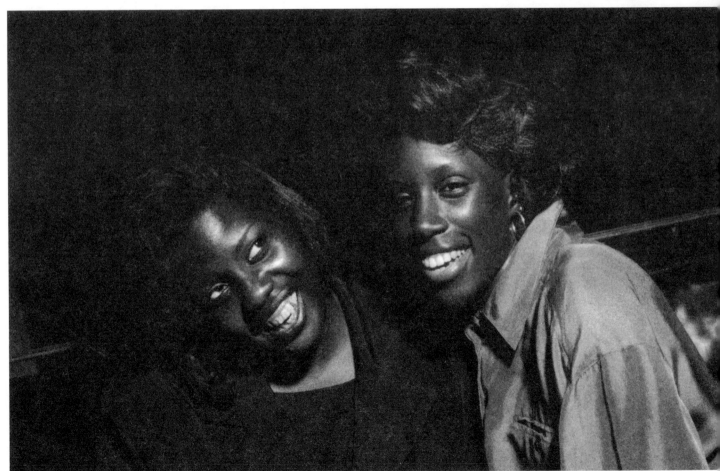

I'm not an old woman
Daphne Jackson, right, with her friend Audrey Haddon-Wilson, went to a seminar on breast cancer and examined a suspicious lump in a silicon breast that was passed around.
worry. She was only 27. "When I had to have a sonogram because they said I was too young for a mammogram, I felt like, 'See, there's not even a question of breast canc

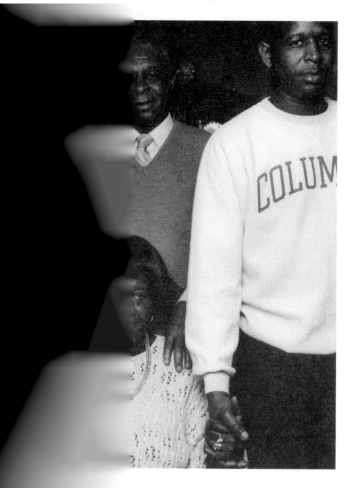

Don't let it swallow you
It has been 22 years since Hermie Gibson had a radical mastectomy. She has been a good Samaritan for other breast cancer victims, with her family at her side. That's daughter Bessie Rhoden, husband John and son Steven. "For me, helping other people is what it's all about. I never let breast cancer surround me—if you do that, it will swallow you up."

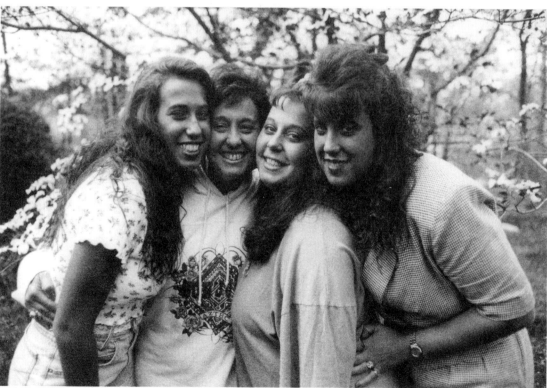

Family matters
Adrienne, Anna, Jennifer and Cynthia Alogna in their backyard. When she had a mastectomy and got laid off, Anna Alogna's life came to a halt. "I lost my whole personality. I looked in the mirror and tried to smile but it's like I'd forgotten how to form one."

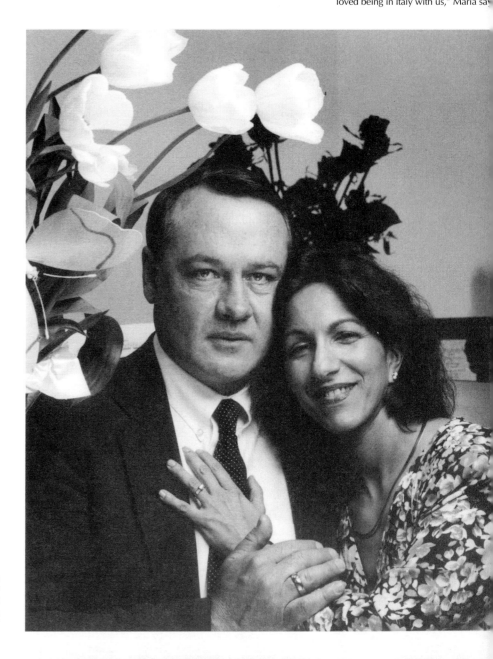

The Florio sist[e]
Jean, Domenica Florio, Maria Bellini a[nd]
Josephine Vojtech at sister Laura's grave[s]
on her birthday. "Laura, we all went to Ita[ly]
in August," Jo says softly. "You would ha[ve]
loved being in Italy with us," Maria say[s]

Life, pass it on
Samuel Scudder and fiance Elise Sobol show off her new
engagement ring. "From the minute I laid eyes on him I
didn't see anything else," she says. "After you've been so
ill, you don't hesitate—you go after what you want."

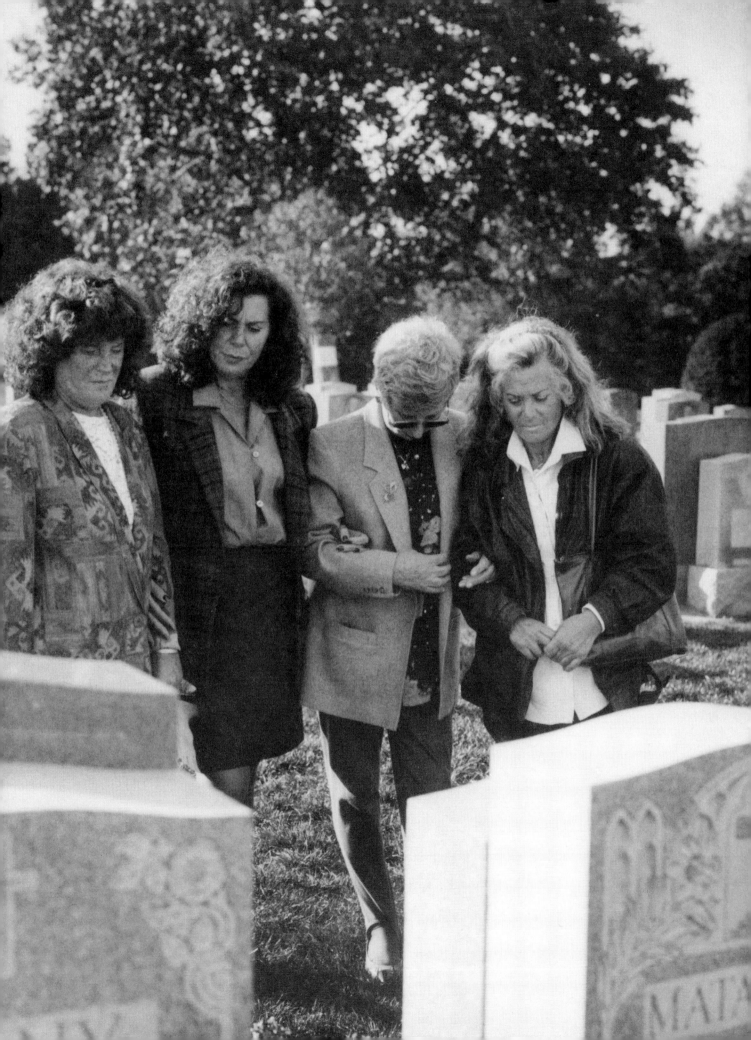

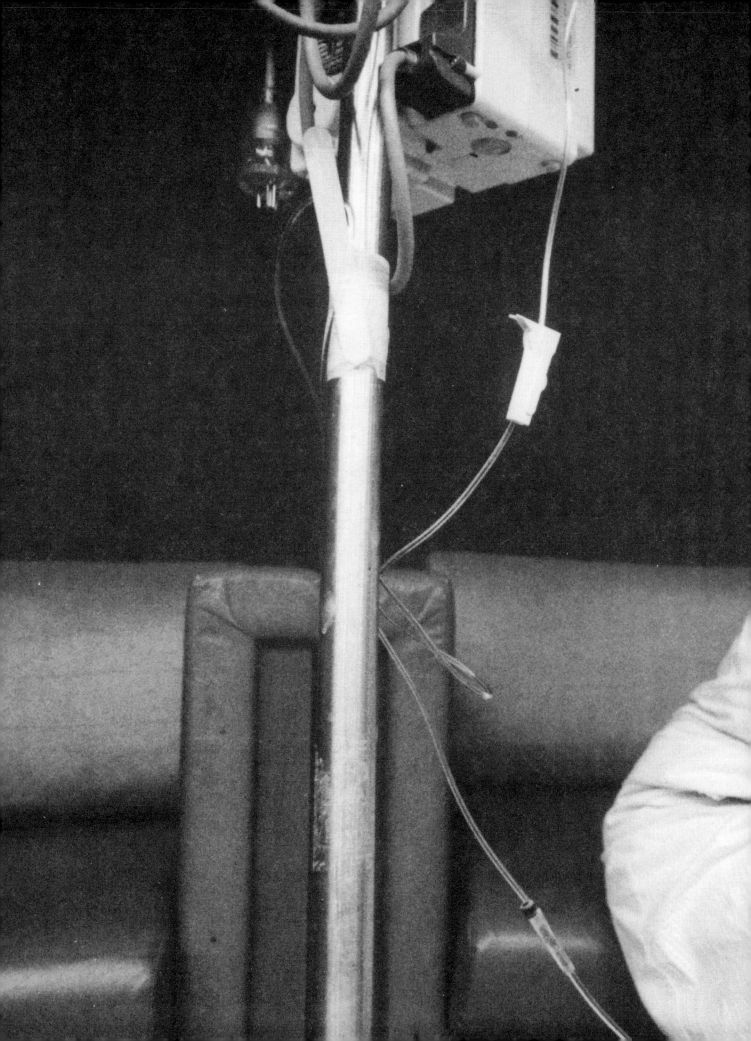

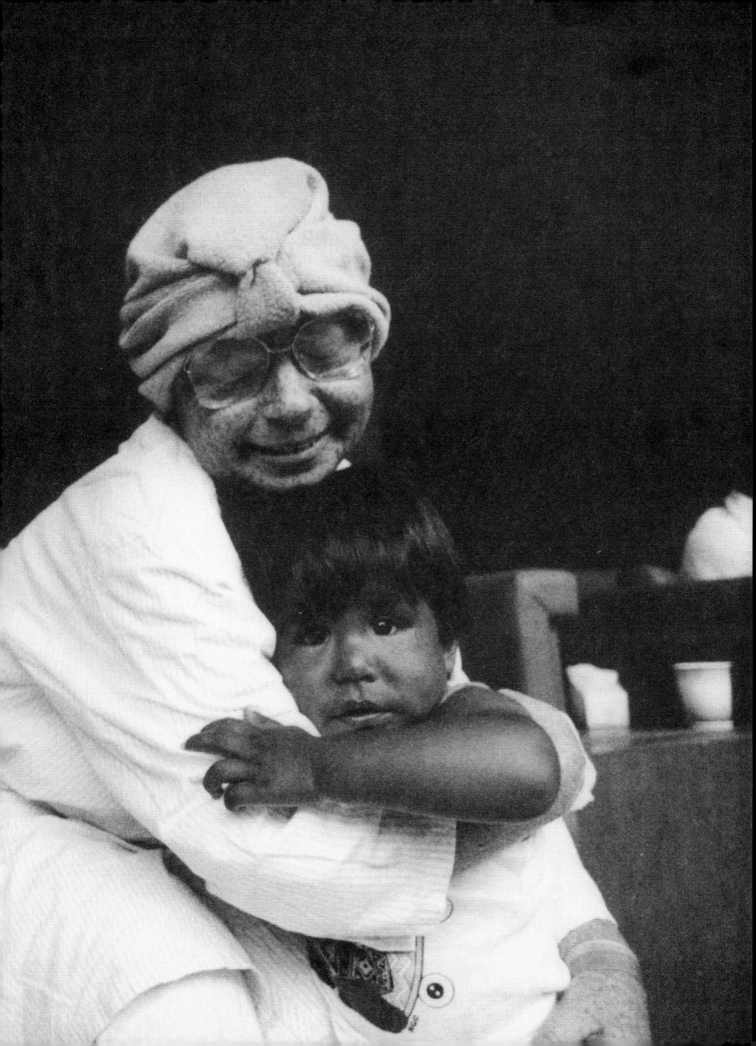

Chemo and a hug
The treatments seem to work better together for Francene Montalbano and son James Vincent Montalbano. After a bone marrow transplant, she was back at work and trying to care for her son. "I'm angry now. How could this happen to me? All we wanted was to be a family."

That's my ha
Her hair is starting to gro back and she usually wears wig, but Thomasine Demt still saves the hair she lo during chemotherapy. "I say, don't care if it's not on n head, that's my hair and I' keeping it.

Sweet victory
When she came home from the hospital after her lumpectomy, Paula Leahy of Smithtown attacked her mammogram with a kitchen knife. She cut out the tumor. Six years later, she still wears a pin over her left breast each day. "I was so proud of my breast. It deserves a medal of honor." She fought a war and has won.

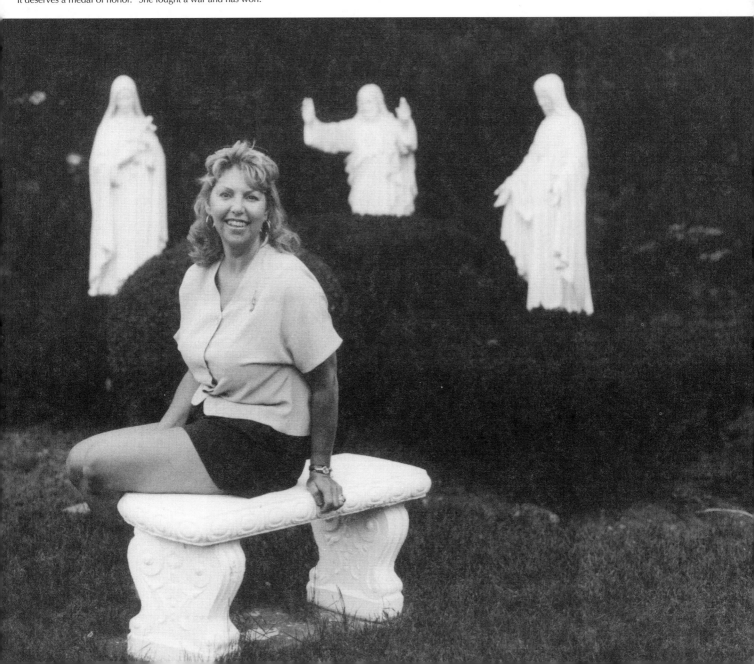

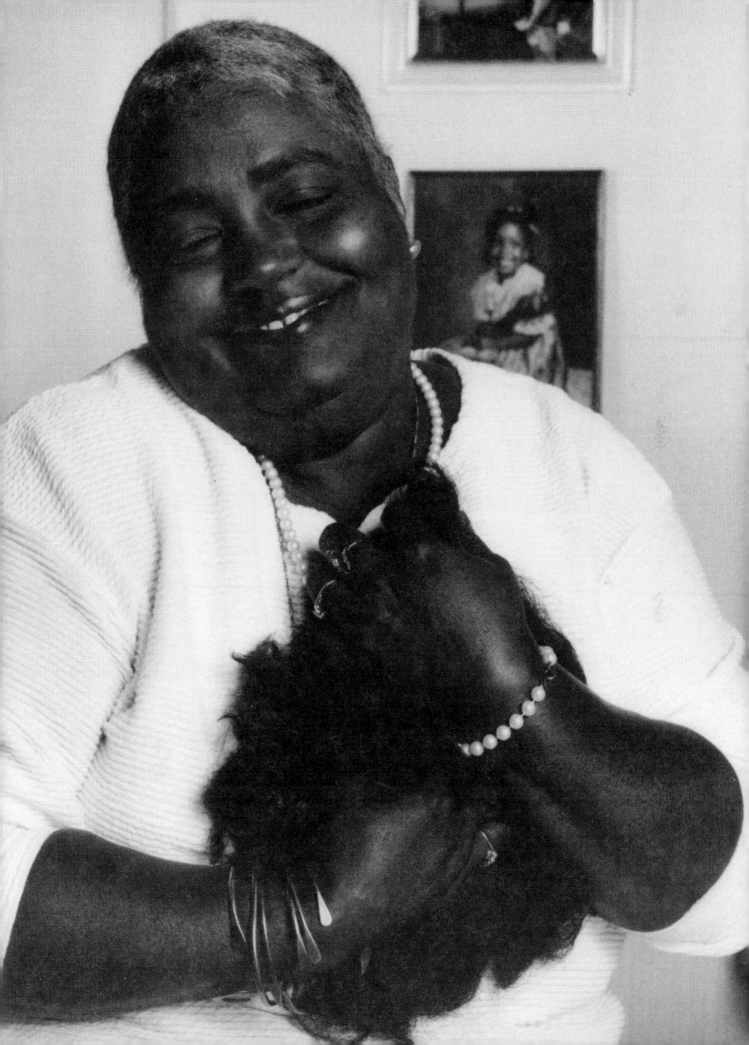

CHAPTER 3

The Fear Never Really Goes Away

There were six of them. Maria, Laura, Faye, Josephine, Jean and Domenica. The Florio sisters.

They were always full of life. As children in Italy, where the girls and their only brother played on their father's farm in Rutigliano, a village just south of Bari, eating the fresh fruits Vito Florio grew on the sun-drenched fields—figs and cherries and grapes and apricots. As teenagers in America, little women in a yellow stucco house on Elm Street in Flushing, Queens, where their mother recreated the old country in the kitchen and the whole family laughed and labored as they struggled to learn the language of their new land. And as wives and mothers, bringing up their own children in Yonkers and New Jersey and on Long Island in Great Neck and Syosset.

Faye was the most outgoing—with a love of life as visible as her dimples. She was a seamstress who made her own dresses and draperies and slip-covers. She loved to dance and she loved to drive—especially in the car her husband, Ed Pezza, bought for her, a white Buick convertible with red interior. They were still young marrieds on the night in 1964 when Ed felt the lump in her right breast. She was only thirty-seven when she died almost ten years later.

Faye was the first of the Florio sisters to get breast cancer.

Laura was two years older than Faye and by all accounts, her mother's favorite. Laura, whose married name was Reda, was the most beautiful sister—with dark wavy hair that cascaded to her shoulders and sparkling eyes and the flawless complexion of a madonna. Laura left her two young sons for a week to nurse Faye after surgery. It is part of Florio family history that Laura and Faye were drinking coffee together one morning when Laura scratched under her left arm and felt a hard knot.

"What's this?" she wondered out loud. "Now, I've got it too?"

Faye didn't laugh. It was just three weeks after her own mastectomy. She touched her sister's lump. "Get yourself to the doctor right away," she said.

More than a decade after her left breast was removed, Laura found a lump in her right breast. She was forty-four when she died on Christmas Day in 1978.

Laura was the second of the Florio sisters to get breast cancer.

Maria is the oldest. Grace and Vito Florio were living with relatives in Queens when Maria, their first child, was born. A year later, when their son Dominick came along, the land of opportunity was in the grip of the Great Depression. The Florio family went home to Italy. When she was seventeen,

Maria recrossed the ocean alone to live with her mother's sister in New York and to etch a new beginning for the others. For four years, she worked in a factory making dress shields so she could save money to help buy the yellow stucco house in Flushing. She married Umberto Bellini, an engineer, and they settled first in Great Neck and then moved east across Long Island to Sag Harbor. Maria never felt a lump. The news showed up on a mammogram. She was fifty-eight and had just become a grandmother.

Maria had a mastectomy and went through six months of chemotherapy. She has been in remission for almost five years.

Maria was the third of the Florio sisters to get breast cancer.

Jean is the second youngest—with auburn hair and a face full of freckles. She was always the shy one. She was the last of the sisters to get her driver's license, the last to become an American citizen, the last to get married. Jean found a lump two weeks before her son's wedding—when she woke up in the middle of the night and rubbed under her right arm.

Like Maria, Jean had a mastectomy and underwent chemotherapy. And like Maria, she lives somewhere between fear and hope. This week Jean marks three years of being cancer-free. But the freedom is conditional. The fear never really goes away, she says. "You think all the time—Will I be okay forever? Will my sisters stay okay? What about my daughters?"

Jean was the fourth of the Florio sisters to get breast cancer.

So far, Domenica, the youngest, and Josephine, who still carries prayer cards from her sisters' funerals in her red wallet, have escaped. But their souls are haunted by the shadow of what all the Florio sisters call the family curse. The shadow hovers in questions that are anything but hypothetical.

Questions without answers.

Will it happen to me, too? When? Why us?

Questions that send Josephine and Domenica to the doctor every six months for a check-up and every year for a mammogram. Questions that have turned Josephine Vojtech into a daily practitioner of breast self-exam. "Every night I put my arms over my head and look in the mirror at my breasts," she says. "I think of Faye and Laura and then I think of Maria and Jean. I'm afraid to examine myself and I'm afraid not to. I feel my heart going boom, boom, boom because I've seen what breast cancer does to you. Before I touch my breasts, I always say a prayer."

This a story of prayers and love and family. Of Faye and Laura, who died. Of Maria and Jean, who survived. Of Domenica and Josephine, who have escaped. A story that spans two continents and generations of women. A story that reaches beyond the six sisters and shadows their daughters and their daughters' daughters. It is, in its most terrible aspect, a story of inheritance.

A story about the power of genetics.

"For me," Jean says, "I don't believe all these things I hear about electric wires and microwaves and blow-dryers. I don't blame the water. I don't blame Long Island. I blame my genes."

The Florio sisters can trace the blame back only one generation—beyond that they have no genealogy of the illness. As far as they can tell, there is no history of breast cancer in their mother's family. Grace Florio outlived two of her children. She survived cancer-free into her eighties, dying of a stroke two years ago. The grim inheritance comes from the paternal side of the family. Vito Florio—a heavy smoker who died of lung cancer in 1971—had a brother and four sisters. Fortunata Calisi, his oldest sister, died in Italy after a seven-year battle with breast cancer shortly after she turned fifty in the 1940s. A granddaughter of Fortunata, also in Italy, died of the disease last year at the age of forty-two. And some family members believe breast cancer killed the two daughters of one of Vito Florio's other sisters.

"I remember Fortunata was a big woman, tall and strong," says Maria, who was about twelve when her aunt died. "It seemed strange to me when all of a sudden my aunt was always in bed. She was sick for a long time. She died at home. Nobody knew Fortunata was only the first. Nobody told us girls we were all in danger. We never thought of it as a family thing back then."

Even when Fortunata's namesake—Faye—got the news of her own cancer, it just seemed like a coincidence. Grace and Vito Florio had named their third daughter after Fortunata, but the namesake became Faye in America. She was a slim young woman who took night school classes and worked days in a Q-tip factory in Queens and fell in love on the assembly line.

The day after her husband felt a lump in her breast, Faye called her sister Josephine, who still remembers the conversation.

"What are you gonna do, Faye?"

"It'll go away. Don't say anything to Ma."

"Go to the doctor, Faye. What does Eddie say?"

"He says go to the doctor."

"Then go."

"We'll see. I think maybe it will go away."

A few days later, Faye called again.

"Guess what Jo? They're going to cut off my breast. They say I have cancer in my breast. Didn't Poppa's sister die of that?"

"Yeah. But she was old. In those years it was different."

"I don't know Jo. I think I'm gonna die just like Aunt Fortunata."

"Don't be silly. You'll be okay. It has nothing to do with Fortunata."

But it did. Experts say ten percent of all breast cancers are inherited—about half of them from a single gene. The Florio sisters seem to fall into this category. Especially the two who died. Jean and Maria, because they were in their fifties when they were diagnosed, are more difficult to classify, according to Dr. Matthew B. Lubin, medical geneticist at Strang Cancer Prevention Center in Manhattan. "When there's a single inherited gene in a family, you see breast cancers at early ages," he explained. "Usually half the people at risk will be affected. Out of these six sisters, four developed the disease—that's pretty close to half. I'd suggest that in this family the father had the gene, which means that all of his daughters had a fifty-fifty chance of getting breast cancer."

If the sisters tried to think Faye's cancer didn't have anything to do with genetics, their mother faced the terror. In the spring of 1964, when she found out Faye needed a mastectomy, Grace Florio held her twenty-eight-year-old daughter in her arms and cried: "Please, no. Not like Fortunata. Dear God, not like Fortunata."

"We were so ignorant then," Jean says now. "To us, it was a fluke that this happened to Faye. We were scared for our sister but it never entered our minds to be scared for ourselves too."

Fear flourished soon afterward when Laura needed a biopsy. On the way to the hospital, Laura drove by the beige, two-story house where her sister Josephine still lives. It was summertime and Jo was watering the flower garden in her front yard. She picked a red-and-yellow rose. "It's as beautiful as you are," Jo told her sister. She handed the flower to Laura. "For good luck."

But the rose faded in the shadow of the family curse. Within a month of one sister's mastectomy, the other sister was undergoing the same surgery. The sisters remember Faye and Laura hugging each other. "So who's gonna die first?" Faye wondered out loud.

"Laura was the wake-up call for the rest of us," says Josephine. "I remember thinking, 'If two sisters could get it, a third one could get it.' I remember lying awake at night wondering, 'Oh boy, who's next?'"

"We're the kind of girls, all of us—we're not criers; we don't get sick worrying," says Maria. "But with Laura, we started to change our attitude."

"We started to get frightened and we started to wonder," says Josephine. "Why our family?"

Laura's doctor told them. "He told us, 'Breast cancer runs in families,'" Jean remembers. "He said, 'You girls better get yourselves checked.'"

They did it together. Maria and Josephine and Jean and Domenica—all of them young mothers, by this time—met at a clinic in Manhattan, where they had their first breast examinations and their first mammograms. No shadows appeared. "I guess somewhere inside we were nervous," says Jean, "but we didn't really expect to get bad news. We took it seriously enough to promise each other that we'd go to our own doctors every year. But we still didn't appreciate how much at risk we all were."

Slowly, as the sisters tried to resume their own lives, they found out. Faye and her family moved to New Jersey and she worked as a seamstress at a dry-cleaners. Josephine dealt with the stress of caring for a retarded son. Maria moved into a center-hall colonial in the well-to-do suburb of Great Neck. Laura visited with her mother every evening over cappuccino. Jean was busy with two toddlers. Domenica gave birth to her second child, a son. But radiation treatments left both Faye and Laura badly burned. And Faye was always in and out of hospitals. As a result of a radical mastectomy, her right arm swelled to four times its normal size, the skin cracked, pus seeped out. She had to keep it tightly wrapped with an Ace bandage and remove fluid from it daily with an electric pump.

Almost a decade after she was diagnosed, in the spring of 1974, Faye Florio Pezza was dying. She underwent more surgery and more radiation treatments. She developed lumps on her head that oozed fluid. She cut off her blond hair. She wore kerchiefs. Ed bought her a wig. Chemotherapy and blood transfusions didn't help. She fought depression. "She'd call up and cry, 'What's happening to me?'" remembers Jean. "'Why is this happening to me?'"

For three months Faye was bedridden. "I was living a lie," recalls Ed. "I told her she looked beautiful. I told her she'd be okay. She wanted to believe me but I think she knew she was dying."

The family held together. Grace Florio came to help; the sisters visited on weekends. Jo cleaned the house. Maria cooked. Domenica sat by her sister's bedside and read Italian magazines to her. Jean watched the children. "Faye loved children," says Jean. "She'd call my four-year-old to her bedside and say 'Recite the alphabet for Aunt Faye.' Until she was bedridden, Faye would think nothing of making her daughter a jumper or skirt just so she'd have something different to wear to school the next day." Laura, who was doing well since her surgery, didn't visit that often. "I think it was too difficult for her to see what was happening," says Ed.

Eventually, Faye was hospitalized. Jean remembers the night a priest came to her sister's room to give her communion. "She asked him, 'Do they have dancing in heaven, Father? If they have dancing, I'm ready; I'll be happy there.'" Maria remembers another night—when Faye was so heavily medicated that she was in and out of consciousness. She hadn't spoken for days. Maria and Laura and their mother sat by her hospital bed. The sisters were arguing. "About something stupid, I can't even remember what," says Maria. "All of a sudden, Faye opened her eyes and said in a clear voice, 'Will you please shut up and stop fighting? Why don't you learn to love each other?' That was the last time I heard Faye's voice. I still feel guilty."

Faye died just before Thanksgiving. She left an eleven-year-old daughter and sons aged thirteen and fifteen. And Ed, who held her like a keepsake in heart and memory. Ed never remarried and lives in Indiana now. He still keeps a picture of Faye on his bureau. "A day doesn't go by that I don't think about my wife," he says. "No one could ever measure up to Faye."

After Faye died, Laura telephoned Josephine. "My God, I'm scared, Jo," she said. "Look at Faye. How much time could I have left?"

"Don't worry. You feel good, Laura. You look good."

"I don't know. I think I'm going to die too."

Then she had the second mastectomy. She consulted a plastic surgeon about silicone implants, which were new at the time. But she'd had two radical mastectomies and there wasn't enough muscle and tissue left. Chemotherapy turned her complexion ruddy and left her lustrous wavy hair frizzy. Then the cancer went to her bones.

Maria visited Laura in the hospital on Christmas Eve, 1978. "She knew she was going. She'd just said good-bye to her two sons. She gave them her wedding and engagement rings and divided her jewelry between them. She told them she loved them. Then she told her husband to take them home. When I left I said, 'I'll see you tomorrow.' When I kissed her goodnight and wished her a Merry Christmas, she squeezed my hand. We got the call the next day that she was gone."

Four years after Faye's death, Laura was buried. And the shadow became a daily companion for the four who were left.

"I don't let myself push the fear away. It's on my mind every day," Josephine says.

Sometimes the fear was palpable. Faye and Laura had just had their mastectomies when Domenica felt lumps in both breasts during a self-exam. The doctor told her the lumps were probably cysts but should be removed. The youngest Florio sister signed a consent form agreeing to a bi-lateral mastectomy if a malignancy was found. "When I came out of anesthesia I touched myself to see if I still had breasts. I couldn't feel anything. My chest was wrapped with bandages. I was crying. I thought, 'I'm number three.' I begged the nurse, 'Please tell me, do I have breasts or don't I?'"

"Yes," the nurse told her. "You have breasts." The cysts were benign. Domenica had escaped.

Josephine came face-to-face with the fear seven years ago when she started menopause. "The glands on the side of my left breast were swollen. I called my gynecologist in a panic. This was in 1986 and Maria and Jean didn't have it yet. I thought, 'Jesus, I'm next.' I went crazy. I went to a specialist in New York City and told him about Faye and Laura. While he was examining me, my husband Jerry went out to put money in the parking meter. The doctor said, 'We'll wait till your husband comes back to talk.'

"I was shaking and sweating. I thought I'd pass out. The doctor was an old man. I thought 'what does he know?' I think I was turning green. Jerry came in and the doctor said, 'Take this young lady and go have a cup of coffee.' He said to me, 'You're going through menopause and your breasts change. It's normal. It's okay. Go have a good dinner, go home and have good sex.'

"I don't have breast cancer? I'm not going to be the next to die?"

"He said, 'No.'

"Doctor can I kiss you?' I asked. I kissed him and we went home and my husband and I had a good lunch, but no sex.

"I called my sisters and we cried with relief."

Relief only lasted two years. In 1988, Maria's mammogram showed a mass in her left breast. "When I heard the doctor say the words 'suspicious' and 'biopsy'

I started to shake," Maria recalls. "My first thought was I'm going to die. Just like Faye and just like Laura. I tried to calm myself but in my heart I knew I was the third sister to have breast cancer."

Maria's husband, Umberto Bellini, was in Italy visiting his parents, so she called her daughter, who'd just given birth to her first child. "At first my mother thought the diagnosis of breast cancer was a death sentence," says Lisa Bellini Gergley, who now lives in California and has a daughter and a son. "How could she not, after what happened with her sisters? She never knew anyone who'd survived breast cancer."

And then Maria called her sisters. She told each of them, "It's starting all over again . . ."

On January 14, 1989, Maria Bellini was the third of the Florio sisters to undergo a mastectomy. Before her surgery, she stood in front of a mirror and said good-bye to her left breast. "It didn't look any different; it didn't feel any different. But I knew it was. I knew they had to cut it off for me to be safe. I said to myself, 'There's a lump in there and it's cancer. The breast has to go. I can't change that. But I can fight the cancer. I'm not Faye. I'm not Laura. I'm Maria. I don't have to die.'"

Not quite two years later, it was Jean's turn.

It was three o'clock in the morning when Jean's sleep was broken by pins-and-needles in her right hand. Half asleep, she shook her arm and massaged it all the way up to her armpit. The lump was hard, about the size of an olive. In an instant Jean was wide awake. She sat on the couch in the dark. At dawn, she went for a walk along the beach in Sag Harbor, where she and her husband have a second home. "I kept touching it and wondering, 'what's this?' But I didn't panic. If it was in my breast I would have been hysterical. My husband told me to go to the doctor. But my son's wedding was two weeks away so it went right out of my mind."

A few weeks later, Jean went for a biopsy. That's when she telephoned her sisters. "Guess what?" she asked Josephine.

"No. It can't be. What is this—are we all going to get it?"

Maria cried when Jean told her. "Not you too. Not again."

Jean had her mastectomy on November 17, 1990. "I didn't let myself think about it because all I did was remember how Faye and Laura looked at the end. I'd try to push them out of my mind and think only about Maria. Maria was in the hospital for a few days. She had six months of chemo but she never got sick, she didn't lose her hair. I prayed and prayed that I'd be lucky like Maria."

And she has been. But like Maria, she keeps her fingers crossed. They all do. Even the ones who have never been touched by the shadow.

Domenica, a hairdresser and mother of two who is going through her second divorce, has a cyst in her left breast and another in her uterus that doctors have been watching for three years. Domenica, who uses her maiden name, insists she'd never have a mastectomy. "When Laura died, it made my insides sick. I shut down and didn't want to hear anything about breast cancer. When Maria got it, I decided that I wasn't going to get close to any of my sisters anymore. I kept my distance emotionally. Now, I'm finally talking about my terror of breast cancer and my fear of losing my sisters."

Josephine has her own incantation. She whispers a prayer before she examines her breasts, then says out loud—"Breast cancer doesn't have to be my destiny."

She just may be right. The older Josephine and Domenica get without developing breast cancer, the better their chances are of remaining free of the disease. "The older they get, the less likely it is that they inherited the gene from their father," explains Dr. Lubin. If so, their daughters and granddaughters may also escape the shadow.

Even so, they have cause to worry. Between the six Florio sisters there are six daughters and eight sons. There are seven granddaughters. And then there are Dominick's three daughters and two granddaughters. Theoretically, all of them could inherit and pass along a gene.

Diana Burchfield—Faye's only daughter who lives in Indiana—evokes the lasting pain of a young mother's breast cancer on her children. "I have photographs of my mother but I can't remember her voice. I can't remember the last time she kissed me goodnight or the last time I told her I loved her. I remember she kept plastic covers on the furniture in the living room and she made me and my brothers brush our teeth before we opened presents on Christmas morning. But what I remember most was that she was in bed all the time."

Diana was eleven when her mother died—a year younger than her own daughter is now. As she reaches for memories, she brushes against fear. "I think of her whenever I exam my breasts. I had my first mammogram last year when I turned thirty and all I thought about was how my mother didn't make it through her thirties."

The family curse haunts Lisa Bellini Gergley, who speaks for her generation and the ones to come. "I'm fearful for my mother and for myself," says Maria's firstborn, at thirty-four the oldest of the Florio sisters' daughters. "And for my daughter. I wanted to name her Laura after my aunt. When I was fourteen, I went to Italy with Laura, my mother and my grandmother. Laura was such fun. She loved the beach and it broke my heart years later when I saw her in the hospital. She was moaning and calling out that she was thirsty. I wet a face cloth and placed it on her lips. I didn't want my daughter to grow up in that memory. I named her Daniela Laura. She's only five but when she's old enough to understand I'll tell her about my aunts and I'll stress that breast cancer is something she must always be aware of.

"I was twenty-nine when my mother was diagnosed. I went to my ob/gyn and explained my family history. I said, 'Tell me what I have to do to prevent this from happening to me.'

"He said, 'Have a mastectomy right now.'

"I was shocked. I said, 'How dare you?'

"He said, 'If you don't have breasts you can't get breast cancer.'

"I said, 'I just had my first baby. I'm breast-feeding. I want more children. Forget it. I'll take my chances.'

"I'm not at all cavalier about it though. I watch myself. I exercise and eat low-fat foods—my husband is an exercise physiologist and I'm a registered dietitian. I have a breast exam every six months. I try to do self-exams in between. I go for a mammogram every year. I had my first mammogram after my mother's surgery. A mass showed up that turned out to be a blocked milk duct. It went away on its own. But I was terrified.

"I was always the one who asked questions. I'd ask my mother, 'Did Faye and Laura eat differently from the rest of the family?' Aunt Faye was so skinny; she was a real Twiggy. I'd ask, 'What did you eat growing up in Italy?' My mother told me about the fresh vegetables and fruits, all homegrown with no pesticides. It's not diet in their case; it's not environmental. I'd ask her, 'Was it the stress of coming from another country?' I'd read that pent-up anger can cause cancer. I asked her, 'Were they angry?' My mother said, 'No, no. Laura loved life. Faye too.' With my family, you can't pinpoint anything from the outside. It's genetic. Which makes it even scarier."

But the Florio sisters still savor life. Domenica goes sailing. Maria winters in Florida with her husband. Josephine takes joy in her flower garden. Jean walks for two hours every morning and goes on business trips to Toronto and San Francisco with her older daughter Jennifer, who organizes direct-marketing conferences. "My mom and her sisters are not bitter about their family history," Jennifer says. "The strength of their acceptance and their ability to move beyond breast cancer is remarkable. Their zest for life is contagious."

Through disease and dispute and even death, through the tugs and tensions of family ties, the Florio sisters stick together. On Christmas Eve they gather at Josephine's two-story house in Bayside, Queens. The next day they share gifts at Jean's sprawling home in Syosset. Thanksgiving is usually at Domenica's place in Sag Harbor. And Easter is always up for grabs. This summer, Maria and Jo and Jean and Domenica went to Italy, to the hometown where they were children together on their father's farm. They look at photographs of the trip and they laugh and talk and remember Faye and Laura.

The trees in St. Mary's Cemetery in Bayside glow amber and red and yellow on a cool clear fall afternoon. Grace Florio would have been eighty-five on this day and the four Florio sisters have come here to sing Happy Birthday at her grave. But first they walk down another row of graves. They stop when they come to a simple granite stone that reads "REDA LAURA 1934 1978 Hail Mary, Pray for Us." There are fading pink geraniums on the grave but the russet and white chrysanthemums are in bloom. The sisters stand together—Jean, Domenica, Maria and Jo—and look at the tombstone. They cross themselves, then hold hands. They whisper "Hail Mary . . ."

Jo speaks first. Like all of the Florio sisters, she still speaks with the musical accent of the land of her childhood. "Laura, we all went to Italy in August."

"We went to the place you loved best," says Domenica. "We went to the island of Ischia and thought of you, Laura."

The tension between the oldest and the youngest crackles like the dried leaves underfoot.

"She knows," says Maria.

"So, I'll tell her anyway," says Domenica.

Jean bends to pinch back the geraniums she planted on Laura's grave for Mother's Day. Jo pulls a few weeds and runs her fingers over the name LAURA. "The flowers came up pretty good for you, Laura. You always loved the flowers."

Domenica places an orange gourd that looks like a miniature pumpkin on the gravestone. She's written "To Laura" on it and drawn a heart and signed her name.

The sisters stand back in a semicircle around the grave.

Jean bows her head. "I remember your smile, Laura. You were always smiling."

Domenica looks off into the distance. "I remember what a wonderful cook you were."

Maria huddles against the wind. "And how beautiful you were."

"I miss you Laura," Jean says.

"A lot," Jo says.

"You would have loved being in Italy with us," says Maria. "I remember how you always wanted to go home to Italy. We laughed so much together. I could hear your laugh. It was like you were right there with us—like we were girls again."

The sisters fall silent and the wind rustles the leaves on the grave. One by one they cross themselves. Domenica says, "Peace be with you always, Laura." Josephine is the last to leave. She stoops in front of the gravestone and places her hand over the name etched in stone. "My sister," she whispers. "I love you."

The day turns colder as Maria and Josephine and Jean and Domenica leave their sister and walk to their mother's grave to sing Happy Birthday. The Florio sisters. Once there were six of them. The four who are left are still full of life.

CHAPTER 4

Elise Sobol: A Survivor

Suddenly last summer, Elise Sobol found herself listening to Samuel Scudder's life story.

It happened minutes after they met at a mutual friend's barbecue. Elise was touched as Samuel told her how he'd married at twenty-five and had a daughter named Stacy Dawn because she was born at daybreak and had bought a three-bedroom house on three-quarters of an acre that he and his wife had scrimped and saved for. How his world was shattered by a pea-size lump that grew as big as a golf ball in his wife's breast before she finally was diagnosed with cancer and had a mastectomy. How her disease spread to her chest wall and pelvis and spine and how he watched her die at home less than two years later, at the age of twenty-six—just a few weeks before their little girl started kindergarten.

Elise heard how he spent the next fourteen years trying to bury his sorrow in work—full time on a Long Island Rail Road maintenance crew and part time in construction and clamming. How he devoted himself to raising Stacy, who was a nineteen-year-old college freshman, and how he'd recently moved back in with his elderly mother.

When Samuel finished, Elise, a forty-two-year-old divorced mother of two, decided her own life story could wait. There was only one overpowering detail that couldn't.

She gulped and then in a steady voice said, "I've had breast cancer."

Neither of them remember the words they spoke afterward, but within weeks Elise and Samuel were dating. Less than a year later, on a day when the crocuses bloomed purple and yellow, they exchanged engagement rings. The rings are fashioned from the diamond wedding band that Elise's grandfather designed for her grandmother almost a century ago. To Elise, that makes them symbols of love and commitment. But they are also symbols of survival. In their own ways, Elise and Samuel are survivors of breast cancer.

"I wasn't looking for anyone to share my life," says the dark-haired piano teacher who met Samuel just months after she underwent a double mastectomy. "I was just happy to have a life. But I shook his hand and it was like *Sleepless in Seattle*. From the minute I laid eyes on him, I didn't see anything else. After you've been so ill, you don't hesitate—you go after what you want."

"I'd been by myself a long time," says Samuel. "I was lonely, but I was resigned in thinking this was the way it would always be. And then this beautiful, wonderful woman walked into my life, and my whole world opened up."

If love walked right in for Elise Sobol, it can never chase all the shadows away.

The shadows had haunted the women in her family for generations—her grandmother died of stomach cancer and an aunt of leukemia. Five years ago, her mother died of breast cancer. Elise went for mammograms every six months. After three years, her doctor suggested she have them on an annual basis. The following year, on Halloween 1993, Elise Sobol was diagnosed with breast cancer. It was an aggressive type of cancer that had already infiltrated much of her left breast—the same type that killed her mother, spreading from the breast to the bones, and eventually the brain, before she was even diagnosed. And to make things worse, Elise's other breast was determined to be precancerous.

After second and third opinions, Elise Sobol consented to a bilateral mastectomy—with her right breast removed as a prophylactic or preventive measure. Relatively few breast cancer patients are confronted with such an extreme measure and even fewer agree to it. But considering her family history, Elise was sure she'd made the right decision.

The cancer was surgically removed. No chemotherapy or radiation was necessary. Like many women, Elise had the first stage of breast reconstruction performed at the time of the mastectomy—a procedure that involved placing an empty sack called a tissue expander behind the pectoralis muscle. Over the course of the next several months, fluid was injected into the sack through a side port to stretch the skin. Four months after the mastectomy, Elise had surgery again to have the expander removed from the right side and a permanent implant or prosthesis put in. She also had a skin graft from the groin to create areolas. Three weeks later, permanent reconstruction of the left breast was performed.

And another reconstruction was going on. Elise was restoring her soul. Three weeks after her mastectomy, she sat down at the Steinway baby grand in her living room and played the first and last movements of the Mozart B-Flat Piano Sonata. She remembers the numbness in her upper arms and the discomfort of the tissue expanders pressing her pectoral muscles. But on that cold night in the winter of 1993 Elise Sobol felt whole again for the first time since the mastectomy, not shattered pieces. She even changed the front porch light. "My personality seems redefined," she wrote in her diary. "There is less holding back of essential emotions. If I am not direct in my dealings, I may not have a second chance. One has to live fully in case tomorrow does not come."

Elise was happy to be back at her job as a music teacher in a school program where her special education students made a 9-foot mural decorated with musical notes that rang out "Having You Back Makes Us Feel Like Singing." She was happy being mom again to thirteen-year-old Marlon and eleven-year-old Aaron, driving them to baseball and soccer practice and staging impromptu family concerts in the living room with Elise on the baby grand and Marlon on drums and Aaron on clarinet.

And then in the spring, at a friend's barbecue, tomorrow came. Elise Sobol met Samuel Scudder.

It was a new beginning in both their lives. Two weeks before, Samuel had broken down at his wife's graveside.

"I'm at the end of my rope," he remembers telling the silent grave. "I need to get on with my life. Please, Claudia, I can't take it any more." He told her how their daughter, who'd kept him going, was an adult now, starting college and a life of her own. He told her he was thinking of taking off for Montana or Australia for a fresh start. "I need to find some happiness in my life."

"Two weeks later Elise fell out of the sky," he says. "I believe my wife had something to do with this."

Marriage lies somewhere in the future—they're not sure when. In the meantime, they think about fate, about the gift of life. About survival.

"Samuel and I, we're both survivors of the breast cancer wars," Elise says. "His loss gave me the courage to cross the bridge and reach out to him. When I took a gulp and told him I'd had breast cancer, too, I knew it would either send him packing or bring him closer. But he looked at my survival as a strength not a weakness, not something he should be afraid of."

"Sometimes it makes my hair stand up to think I'm involved with someone who's had breast cancer," Samuel says. "I mean, my wife's passing took away half my world. But I looked at Elise and thought wow. I know exactly what she's been through, the kind of strength it takes to battle this disease. Because of that I can look beyond the surface in a way that maybe other men can't. I never just saw a woman who's had breast cancer. I saw Elise."

"I've been through the war," Elise Sobol says. "But as scarred as I am, I have a new life. I have a future."

ELISE SOBOL: I'm part of a continuum. I have my mother's drive, her ambition, her joy in living—and I also have her breast cancer. When I was diagnosed, I told myself: "Just because your mother died of breast cancer doesn't mean you're going to die of it. Just concentrate on doing what you have to do to get it out of your body."

Every doctor I went to told me the same thing—considering the aggressive nature of your cancer and your family history, you'll probably have to do something about your right breast within a year. The more I thought about it, the more I thought about my mother. My mother never had a chance. Her breast cancer spread before it was even discovered. I didn't want to spend a year of my life worrying and wondering—that's not my style. So I said yes to having my right breast removed as a prophylactic measure. I have no doubts I did the right thing.

I was taught by my mother to face things head on and that's what I did during my passage through cancer. I thank her for teaching me this important lesson. I watched this heroic woman deal with her disease and in her dying she showed me how to live. Cancer has taught me not to be afraid of anything.

———

Anna Alonga: A Survivor

After she had a lumpectomy and started chemotherapy, Anna Alogna got laid off from her job as a bookkeeper. It was too much trouble too fast and she sat in her home and came to a halt.

"I sank into a black hole of depression," she says.

She hardly ate, she stopped cooking for her family, she just looked out her living room window and cried. "I lost my whole personality. I looked in the mirror and tried to smile but it's like I'd forgotten how to form one."

Her children wanted the smile back. More than that, they wanted to see Anna again. One afternoon in March of 1993, the mother and her three daughters found themselves drinking coffee around the kitchen table. Jennifer, the oldest at twenty-two, hugged her mother. "We miss you, Mom."

Anna started to cry.

"We need you, Mom," said Adrienne, the eighteen-year-old.

"We want our mommy back," said seventeen-year-old Cynthia.

"I'm trying," Anna said. "I'm trying."

And then they all cried.

About four months later, Cynthia was hospitalized with depression and Anna Alogna tried harder. She opened her eyes to the world that mattered most, the world encompassed by the four-bedroom colonial on a hill. As if someone were breathing life into her, she started coming back. She had a constant goad— her depression was affecting her family. "I felt like I was losing my family. A happy family was falling apart."

And the only way she could save them was to save herself.

In March of 1991, at the age of forty-two, Anna Alogna went for her first mammogram. She'd never felt better—she was walking three miles a day and eating a low-fat diet. Even though three of her father's four sisters had died of breast cancer, Anna didn't think she had anything to worry about. The exam reassured her. Everything checked out fine.

But by midsummer the following year, Anna was troubled by a soreness above her right breast. And almost every night, she'd awake with the same eerie dream. Her three aunts—Vinnie, Jennie and Mary—hovered around her. They said nothing, they just kept watching her with mournful eyes. By September the pain in Anna's breast was so bad that on a trip to Montauk with her husband,

Iggy, to celebrate their twenty-second anniversary, it hurt her to walk against the wind on the beach.

One night she woke up crying from the intense pain shooting down her right arm. The next morning when she took a shower, Anna did a breast self-exam and felt a lump almost the size of a golf ball. She ran to a gynecologist. "I was white as a ghost, in a total panic but he was very nonchalant about it. He said it was a cyst, that cancer isn't painful. He said, 'If it bothers you we'll aspirate it.'"

Then as suddenly as the pain had started, it disappeared. By now it was almost Christmas and even though Anna noticed that the lump was getting bigger she didn't worry. "I had enough to worry about. It was the holidays, we were re-doing the bathroom, I was working full time. I pushed it off."

She stopped pushing it away when a co-worker was diagnosed with breast cancer. Shaken, Anna called the doctor again. He suggested another mammogram and a sonogram. In the two weeks she had to wait for an appointment, her breast became red and swollen and bumpy. The radiologist took one look at it and referred her to a surgeon. This time the diagnosis was breast cancer.

"It was like being hit over the head with a bat. I became a zombie."

On February 13, 1992, at Mather Memorial Hospital in Port Jefferson, Anna Alogna underwent a lumpectomy—a less disfiguring operation than mastectomy in which the tumor, but not the breast, is removed. The almost-golf-ball-sized lump in Anna's breast turned out to be a four-and-a-half-centimeter tumor. Three weeks later, she had surgery to remove eighteen lymph nodes—eight of which were malignant.

"I tried to pull myself together. I was so relieved I'd had the option of a lumpectomy. My husband said, 'Even if you'd had a mastectomy I'd love you anyway.' But I wasn't sure I'd have loved me anyway. Having the lumpectomy was good for my psyche. I still felt normal."

About a month after her surgery, Anna started chemotherapy. After her first treatment, she realized she'd lose her hair but thanks to anti-nausea drugs, she wouldn't necessarily be sick. It was April and she decided it was time to go back to her job as a bookkeeper for a nonprofit organization. Her supervisor told her that the agency no longer needed her.

"Is it because I have breast cancer?" Anna asked.

"No. No," she remembers the supervisor insisting. "We have volunteers to do your job."

Anna wound up with two weeks of vacation pay and two months of severance pay. "In my heart I know they took my job away because I had breast cancer. I've decided it's not worth aggravating myself over. It's on their conscience. But what they really did was knock me out of the ballpark, emotionally speaking."

Throughout the rest of 1992 and into the following year, a woman's life came to a complete halt. The energetic woman with a Brooklyn accent who was always up by six in the morning to make breakfast for her husband, the matriarch of her family who was known for her ravioli and her chicken cutlets and her good advice, whose full-time job helped support the two-story house with three bath-rooms, simply disappeared. A different Anna—a thin woman with sallow skin and sunken eyes and no eyelashes—wandered the house in her nightgown. She'd stare out the window for hours or lay on her bed and cry. "I felt like I was losing everything, myself, my future. All I could think was, 'How will I ever be like I was? I'm going to die like my aunts.'"

Sometimes, Anna would hear Cynthia crying in her room. She'd sit on her youngest daughter's bed and ask what's wrong. "Mommy, I'm so scared," the teenager would say.

Anna didn't know how to comfort her. "I'm scared, too," she would answer.

Cynthia, a high school sophomore at the time, took her mother's breast cancer the hardest.

"I was used to looking to Mommy for advice," says Cynthia, "and all of a sudden she was crying on my shoulders. She'd turn to me and ask me, 'Am I going to die?' She didn't want to face the world. She was afraid we'd lose the house. She was scared like a little girl. She'd sit in a corner and twiddle her fingers or she'd be on the couch rolled up like a ball. I was afraid of losing her but I didn't want her to know. I held it in. My dad was quiet, you couldn't talk to him, he was my mother's backbone but he was a nervous wreck. He'd say, 'Leave Mommy alone.' When I was in school and my mom wasn't there so I didn't have to smile and try to make her happy, that's when I'd feel myself collapsing. I'd leave class and go to a place called the Time Out Room, where kids who are having problems can go to talk to someone. I'd go a couple of times a day."

Anna's depression spread through the family. Iggy—a high school groundskeeper who took his wife to every chemo appointment—pleaded with her, "Please Anna, just talk to me." Jennifer—a data entry clerk who cooked supper for the family every night—tried to drag her mother out for lunch or breakfast. Adrienne—who was in her first year at community college—let her grades take a nose-dive. And the three sisters fought a lot. "We were all so tense trying to cheer Mommy up that we'd explode with each other over a hair clip," Cynthia remembers.

"Somewhere inside me, I knew Cynthia was the one who was really in trouble," Anna says, "but I wasn't sure what to do about it."

There was more reason for sadness. Anna's mother died. And the mother of one of Cynthia's friends died of breast cancer. But Anna was trying and an analogy formed in her mind. An analogy that led to a family's survival. "It's like when you're on an airplane and they tell you the safety procedures—they always say to put your oxygen mask on first and then assist your child. I realized if I'm not okay I can't help my child. So I joined a support group so I could get strong enough to help my daughter."

Anna had been to only one or two meetings of the support group—"mostly I just listened"—when the family was stricken with a new crisis. It hap-pened at night about four months after the daughters talked to their mother in the kitchen. Cynthia took a bunch of tranquilizers and prescription medicines

40

and Advils. "I wanted people to know how depressed I was," she says. "I was so sick of holding everything in. It was late at night and I was talking on the intercom to my friend across the street. I was getting groggy and I told her what I'd done. She called a friend who called my boyfriend who called my dad who called the ambulance. I was in the hospital for three weeks. They put me on Prozac. They said I was depressed and needed to let it out."

That was last summer. Since then, Anna Alogna has returned to her family. Slowly, she learned to let out her fears in her support group and when she bounced back, so did her youngest daughter. It helped when Anna got a part-time job last summer as a data entry clerk for the town street-lighting department.

Now, Anna—whose dark straight hair grew in curly—walks three miles a day and works out at the gym four times a week with her husband. Cynthia is about to graduate from high school. Jennifer has a new job with Suffolk County and Adrienne's grades are back up. Last month for Mother's Day, Anna's three daughters gave her a card that said, "Welcome back, Mom."

"We have our mommy back," Cynthia says, "and everyone's happy now."

"I thought I'd never be happy again. But I am," says Anna. "Something awful came and hit us on the head. But I'm alive and my family survived. Now I say, 'I had breast cancer. I had breast cancer but I'm alive'—and best of all I have my smile back."

ANNA ALOGNA: I told my mother I had a lump removed but not that it was breast cancer. She was in her eighties and I didn't want to give her any more heartache than she'd had in her life. My father was hit and killed by a van in 1973 just after he'd retired and they were starting to enjoy life. Then thirteen years later, both my brother's daughter and my sister's daughter were killed by a drunk driver. I was her baby and I wanted to spare her. She came to stay with us for two weeks when I was going through chemo. It was July and I worried about how I was going to keep this wig on all day. I hated wearing it. It was so hot. The first time she saw me she did a double-take but I told her I'd gotten a perm. In the morning my daughters would tell me, "Grandma's up," and I'd run for my wig. I was sitting at the breakfast table one day and it was so hot and my blood counts were very low. I was dizzy and I leaned back in my chair and just passed out cold. The chair fell back with me in it and my wig went sailing. When I came to, we laughed and cried at the same time. I grabbed for my hair and told her I was on medication for an infection. Later, she told me, "If I didn't die at the sight of you that day, Anna, I'll live forever." I think she must have known the truth. She died last year and I'm glad I never said the words "breast cancer" to her.

Francene Montalbano: A Survivor

Most of the time Francene Montalbano takes things one step at a time. But every now and then, she stops and sits in a chair and cries.

She weeps for all the things she can never have again. In the whisper of a single year, Francene Montalbano lost her husband, her left breast and her home. And for three tortuous months while she lay in a hospital bed, the woman who waited for years to have a child lost her ability to be a mother to her adopted baby boy.

Her saga of loss started in the summer of 1992 in a white Cape Cod where a nursery was decorated with teddy bears and a border of blue sailboats. That spring, Francene, a social worker at an occupational high school for special education students, and her husband James, a librarian, had finally filled the nursery. Francene was forty-four; James was thirty-nine. For much of their marriage they had tried to have a child—James underwent surgery and hormone therapy to correct his low sperm count; Francene took high doses of fertility drugs to enhance her egg production. But nothing worked.

And then just before Easter—on their sixth wedding anniversary—they flew to Guadalajara, Mexico, and adopted a dark-haired, six-week-old infant they named James Vincent Montalbano. "The birth mother was so sweet; she kept saying, 'I love my baby. God bless you for taking my baby,'" Francene remembers. "Her name was Anna Rosa and she was the oldest of nine children. She was just a child herself and we felt like adopting her, too. The day after the adoption, the sewers exploded and Guadalajara was being closed. Our lawyer drove us to the airport on unpaved back roads. We caught the last plane to Mexico City. It was like something out of an adventure movie."

A movie about paradise found. Before they left Mexico, James Montalbano told his wife, "I don't care what the future holds—this little boy has made me feel like a father."

Three months later, Francene felt a lump in her left breast. Her gynecologist advised her to have her first mammogram. But she was too busy and too happy to bother making the appointment. There was a christening party on the covered deck of the white Cape in Lindenhurst, a blue-collar community on the Island's south shore, where the baby they'd nicknamed Jaime wore a white suit from his native land. There was a vacation in the Poconos and excursions to pick apples and pumpkins. And then there was Halloween—and the new parents dressed their baby as a penguin and took him trick-or-treating in a carriage.

If a shadow had fallen across paradise, neither Francene nor James was about to acknowledge its presence.

By late autumn, they didn't have much choice. Francene had a constantly worsening cough and James had chronic stomach pains. James went to the doctor first. Just before Thanksgiving, he was diagnosed with a rare cancer of the outer stomach lining. He would require surgery and chemotherapy but he might be able to live as long as ten years, the doctors told him.

During one of James' early checkups, Francene asked his doctor to prescribe medicine for her cough. Instead, he gave her a physical. "He examined my breast and I saw his face drop."

"I want you to get a mammogram today and see a breast surgeon for a biopsy," Francene remembers the doctor saying.

"I don't have time."

"Make time."

Just weeks after her husband was diagnosed with stomach cancer, Francene Montalbano was diagnosed with breast cancer. On December 8, 1992, her left breast was removed and life took on new definitions. Mastectomy. Chemotherapy. CAT scans. MUGGA scans. Bone marrow transplant. The day James' CAT scan showed spots on his lung, a pathology report showed that all of the twenty-four lymph nodes removed during Francene's mastectomy were malignant. "The look in the doctors' eyes said it all—they looked at me like I was a dead woman."

A bone marrow transplant was recommended but Francene put it on hold because of her husband's worsening condition. She kept it on hold even when additional tests showed a shadow on her lung that darkened her prognosis. The spread of her cancer put Francene into stage four of the disease—with only a ten percent chance of surviving five years.

Parents and child spent Christmas with Francene's sister and her family in Stony Brook. Her sister, Rosemary Cottone, had to buy the presents that Francene and James gave each other and the baby. The school where Francene's brother is a teacher delivered toys from Santa Claus. Out of the hospital briefly after a lung biopsy, James helped choose and decorate the tree. They videotaped their only Christmas together as a family. "I kept thinking next Christmas everything will be better," Francene says, "but there was no next Christmas."

Near the end of January, James lay dying at Memorial Sloan-Kettering Cancer Center in Manhattan. Because of the shadow on her lung, Francene's bone marrow transplant was delayed and she started conventional chemotherapy. Each night for three weeks, she slept on a recliner in James' hospital room. "I tried to hold myself together so I could comfort him in his last days. I knew I was about to become a widow. I couldn't deal with the idea of losing my husband and battling for my own life. My only thought was to be there for Jim."

On February 11, 1993—less than one month after his fortieth birthday—James Montalbano died. Francene wore the purple suit she'd gotten for Christmas to his funeral mass. Hours after she buried her husband, she was at Sloan-Kettering with a 102-degree fever. "Please keep me alive," she begged her doctor. "My baby doesn't have a father now. My baby needs me—he needs his mother."

She needed to be needed. One month after her husband's death, Francene was bald from chemotherapy but she put a Barney hat over her terry-cloth turban and helped her son blow out his birthday candle. By this time, she'd put a "For Sale" sign on her house and moved in with her sister's family. Every night she'd cradle her baby in a bedroom decorated with trucks and trains and a tapestry from Mexico. And when he'd whisper, "Where's Dada?" she'd sit in the dark and sob.

After four months of chemotherapy, the spot on Francene's lung disappeared. It was time for the arduous procedure of high-dose chemotherapy with peripheral stem cell support, a variation on a treatment commonly referred to as bone marrow transplant. A procedure that involves filtering from the bloodstream countless stem cells—the mother cells that give rise to platelets and red and white blood cells. The stem cells are removed and frozen to protect them from the high doses of chemotherapy administered to attack the cancer. Then they are thawed and reintroduced to the body to grow back into the bone marrow and foster the growth of new blood cells.

In almost four years, 112 women—including Francene—have undergone this procedure at Sloan-Kettering. "Most patients who relapse do so within the first year-and-a-half, so for Francene it's too early to tell," said Dr. George Raptis, head of the Sloan program. "But she's closely monitored and there's no evidence of any new changes. Despite all she'd been through, she turned out to be very aggressive in making decisions about herself. I like to think that a patient's attitude helps her get through the treatment and might even affect the outcome. Francene's attitude was very powerful, very strong."

Francene spent most of last summer on the twelfth floor of Sloan-Kettering—fighting infections, shaking with chills, spiking fevers as high as 104 degrees, undergoing dozens of transfusions. She lost forty pounds. "It was hard enough being in the hospital where my husband died but now I had to face the very real possibility of my own death. It crossed my mind that maybe I shouldn't even try to be a mother—maybe I should give Jaime up for adoption. But then I'd hear his voice."

"Where are you, Mama?" a little boy would ask when she telephoned from the hospital.

"Mama misses you," she'd answer.

When Francene was up to it, her sister brought Jaime to visit. "I never realized a baby could be depressed," says Rosemary Cottone, a teacher who has a three-year-old daughter and is eight months pregnant. "Jaime didn't smile, he wouldn't talk, I'd hear him whimpering at night. But when I took him to visit Fran—well, he was a different child as soon as he saw his mama."

Jaime would crawl all over his mother and rest his head in her lap. And Francene would remember what her husband had said about how a little boy had made him feel like a father. "I'd think how lucky I am to have had the chance to hear a baby call me mama."

By summer's end, Francene was back in Stony Brook. She celebrated her forty-fifth birthday a few days later and a dark-haired little boy with chubby cheeks helped his mama blow out her candles.

Since then, Francene Montalbano has been taking things one step at a time. Her fire-engine-red hair has grown back darker and finer and curlier. She's working full-time at a vocational training center although she's cut down her caseload. She's sold the white Cape Cod and looks forward to the extra bedroom and bath her brother-in-law is building for her in his home. "It was hard to let go of my house—it's a symbol of a part of our lives. We just wanted to be a family."

For Francene—and more especially for her son—family has a new meaning. Jaime calls his adopted mother mama—and he calls his aunt and uncle mommy and daddy. "My sister sees Jaime as her own and that's the way I want it," Francene says. "I want him to feel he's part of her family."

"Jaime knows who his mother is," says Rosemary Cottone. "He won't hug or kiss me when his mama is around. And I back off totally when Fran's home. Everyday, I see my sister healing. She's laughing again—she looks full of life—and she's talking about the future. Selling the house was an important closure. And she's starting to get angry. That's good—she has a lot to be angry about."

These days, every step forward that Francene Montalbano takes is a giant step. "I pray the worst is behind me," she says. "I'm not brave—I'm numb. I don't feel strong—I feel battered. I'm just putting one foot in front of the other, trying my best to keep walking forward. What else can I do?"

> *FRANCENE MONTALBANO: I'd like to fly away and start a new life. I'd like to buy a condo and travel. At some point in the future, I'd like to start dating again, maybe remarry and be a family again. But always in the back of my head there's this little voice saying, "But Francene, you have cancer." I mean, who's gonna take this old bag with breast cancer? I'd like to forget the past year, but it keeps hitting me. I'm angry now. How could this happen to me? All we wanted was to be a family. Sometimes, I feel immobilized—I sit like a lump and I cry. I try so hard to figure it all out. I should have appreciated the moment more. I realize now that you really don't have the future—all you have is right now.*

CHAPTER 5

"How Do I Say Good-bye to Jesse?"

The esplanade stretches down West Hudson Street in Long Beach, a mile-long divider of green grass dotted by a few trees and shrubs—and by a single patch that brightens in spring and survives into fall. A rectangle of color that is reborn each year in a splash of purple crocuses and a parade of red tulips and ends in an explosion of gold and crimson chrysanthemums.

The garden grows across the street from the two-story beige-shingled home where Sue Rosenbaum spent most of her adult life. It is the garden she planted herself on city land, running hoses across the road and carrying spades and shears and shovels to build a brick border and turn the hard brown earth and nurture the blossoms.

On a cloudy autumn afternoon Sue Rosenbaum's family and friends huddle against the wind that rustles the red and fuchsia impatiens surviving past their season. It is two days after her death, and the people who love her have come to the garden a few miles from the Atlantic Ocean to say good-bye.

Marc Rosenbaum, Sue's husband, holds their three-year-old daughter in his arms while a minister reads a poem and offers a prayer. Jesse squirms and pinches her father's nose. She giggles and plays with a pink-and-black button pinned over his heart. A button that Sue Rosenbaum kept fastened to the windowpane near her bed, that stayed there like an epitaph during the seemingly endless weeks of her dying.

A button with a simple message—Stop Breast Cancer.

Jesse crawls down from her father's embrace. She runs on tiptoes the way she always does, the way that made her mother laugh and call out, "Jesse Bessie, my beautiful ballerina." She runs to the edge of the garden and picks a gold-colored chrysanthemum that she gives to her father.

"Mommy's flower," Jesse says.

She tip-toes off again, giggling. "I'm picking Mommy's flowers for you," she calls to her father. She comes back with a white chrysanthemum, then lavender, then crimson, then white again. By the time the service ends, Marc Rosenbaum has a bouquet in his hand.

Jesse crawls back into her father's arms. "Don't cry daddy. You have Mommy's flowers. Mommy's flowers are happy."

If she were there, Sue Rosenbaum might have smiled her wonderful smile. "Jesse Bessie," she might have said. "Come here, munchkin." And then she might have broken into her big laugh—the laugh that could still be heard through the final months of her life.

Last Christmas, Sue Rosenbaum asked her mother to put together a photo album of her childhood as a keepsake for Jesse. The first snapshot shows a sleeping baby in a carriage making a fist. "Susan Ellen," the hand-written caption reads, "3 weeks." Flip the pages and she's two years old, digging in the yard of her home in Bethpage. She's four in a cowgirl outfit, complete with hat and holstered six-shooter. She's five in a checkered bathing suit at Jones Beach with her father. At eleven, she stands long-legged in the front yard holding a basketball. And perhaps the most revealing is the photo taken on her twelfth birthday. She models a striped shirtwaist dress with a Peter Pan collar and shows off an equally new baseball mitt. "She wanted that dress the worst way," says her mother, Irene Lord, who now lives upstate with Sue's father. "And oh boy, she wanted that mitt even more. She really wanted that mitt."

In Sue's view of the world, the combination was not incongruous. She had her own style. She did things her way. Susan Ellen Lord was a gymnast and a cheerleader at Bethpage High School. She had a gift for painting. She was skilled at sewing and made her own pink satin gown for the senior prom—she didn't finish the sleeves and the shawl till the night before.

The lanky teenager grew into a joyful woman who loved to dance. That was the way she approached the future. For as long as she could, Sue Rosenbaum made a partner out of life and danced it around the room.

If she was going to make a mistake, it would be hers to make. When she was eighteen, she decided to leave home. There was an argument; it was the first time Sue ever saw her father, a carpenter and volunteer firefighter, cry.

"You don't want to obey the rules, get out," Bill Lord shouted.

"Okay, I'm getting out," Sue shouted back.

Sue was falling in love with a married man, a co-worker in the shoe department of a discount store. He got a divorce and they got married. Neither the bride nor the groom's family attended the civil ceremony. Soon afterward, a daughter, Naomi, was born, and eventually the family wound up in the house in Long Beach. Sue's two stepchildren came to stay with them every weekend.

She helped her husband form his own audio firm, but it wasn't enough. Sue wanted to be more than an at-home mom in a supporting role. Her husband didn't want her to work. So she started painting lessons and blossomed as an artist. And as her marriage fell apart, she wasn't afraid to confide in a young single neighbor named Marc Rosenbaum.

"He was the boy next door," Sue would explain. "He's six years younger than I am, and for years it was just 'Hi neighbor.' But life is funny. We got to be friends, and by the time I was divorced Marc had his own apartment and we were dating."

The divorce came in 1980, after ten years of marriage. Sue and Marc got engaged six years later. This time, everyone attended the wedding. The bride and groom arrived at the synagogue in a white Rolls-Royce. Sue had converted to Judaism in her first marriage, and Marc stepped on a glass at the end of the ceremony—an age-old rite that has come to mean good luck but that symbolizes the fragility of life. The bride carried calla lilies, her favorite flower. She filled baskets with pots of pink and white impatiens as favors for the guests. Sue and Marc played the garter scene with gusto and fed each other wedding cake and danced to a song called "Almost Paradise."

Four years later, Sue thumbed her nose at convention again. When she was thirty-nine she gave birth to her second daughter, Jessica Leigh. "We were happy before Jesse, but we were ecstatic after," Marc says.

"Sue's life fell into place with Marc," her mother says. They had a baby to love and a house to keep fixing up. When they were married, Marc was driving his father's cab in New York City. Sue was pleased when he got a safer job servicing fire extinguishers. She established her own bookkeeping business, working from an office at home. There were birthday parties and holidays, visits to grandma and grandpa upstate, trips to Florida and Maine.

Sue Rosenbaum was living life her way. That was always her goal—even when she was diagnosed with breast cancer.

In April of 1993—on a morning defined by the daffodils and irises opening in the esplanade across the street and blossoming in her yard—Sue Rosenbaum sits at her kitchen table and talks about the summer day almost two years before when she found out that in all likelihood she would die of breast cancer.

That May, she had found the lump in her left breast during a self-exam in the shower. Her gynecologist told her it was just a thickening because she was having her period. A few weeks later her left armpit was sore. The doctor still thought the lump was a thickening but referred her to a general surgeon. The surgeon ordered a mammogram and when nothing showed up, he ordered a sonogram. This time, the lump was labeled suspicious.

Sue still didn't think it was an emergency. She had no family history of the disease, no known risk factors. "I never gave breast cancer a moment's thought."

But she needed a second opinion for insurance purposes, so she consulted a breast specialist. By now it was July and her collarbone was sore and swollen. A biopsy was performed—and Sue Rosenbaum found out she had breast cancer. She tried to take it in stride. "I figured, what the heck, Betty Ford had it, Nancy Reagan had it. I can handle this. I knew so little."

The next day was July 17, 1991, and Sue made a phone call to an oncologist that she would replay for the rest of her life.

"My sister-in-law had mentioned that there were stages of breast cancer, so that was my first question—'What stage am I in?'

"'Stage four,' the doctor said.

"In my head I'm thinking, well, that's not too bad. And so I asked him,—'How many stages are there—ten? twelve?'

"'No,' he said. 'Four.'

"'Are we talking a time period here?' I asked.

"Six months to a year if the chemo doesn't work."

Her cancer was too advanced—it had spread into her lymph system and her collarbone; no further surgery was recommended. She was forty years old. She had just helped her baby daughter blow out the candles on her first birthday cake.

Sue looks out the greenhouse window vibrant with herbs and aloe vera and a donkey-tail cactus. She picks up the story. "A few seconds later, the doctor asked me for the name of my pharmacy so he could order chemo drugs. I hung up the phone and started screaming. My parents and my sister were over, and I told them, 'I have stage-four breast cancer, and I'm going to die.' I beeped Marc to come home. He didn't ask why, he just said, 'I'm on my way.' That's when I really lost it. Total hysteria. I had the babysitter take Jesse to the beach to get her out of the house. When Marc came home he was so upset he was throwing things and cursing."

Two days after the biopsy, Sue was in the Manhattan office of another oncologist, Dr. Ezra Greenspan, a pioneer in the field who is known to colleagues as the father of chemotherapy. She had her first chemo session—a heavy dosage of five drugs that would be repeated twice a week for months. Three weeks later, she lost her hair. Sue cried in her mother's arms. "I'm so ugly, Mom. I feel like an alien, like E.T. I'm bald with dark circles under my eyes. Mom, I look like Uncle Fester from "The Addams Family.""

But just a few weeks later, Sue trudged across the street with a spade and started the garden in the esplanade. She planted pink and white climbing roses and a red azalea. Sue was in a support group, and in the months that followed she planted a crab apple tree and a dogwood and a few evergreens—she planted something every time a friend died. "What am I doing," she told Marc when she came in from the garden one day, "planting a forest out there?"

For the rest of that year and all of 1992, Sue underwent chemotherapy that tapered down to once a week, then every other week. By Christmas, she was going every seven weeks and the sessions had become her security blanket. "I felt safe—as long as I was getting chemo the cancer was being killed."

And then one February morning she woke up with a headache that lasted for days. The headache kept coming back—an intense pressure behind the eyes. Finally, she called Greenspan. "I want you to go for a brain scan," he said.

That same night, Marc took his wife to a local lab. When the test was over, the nurse wouldn't answer her questions. "I put in a call to your doctor," the nurse told her.

"I knew what that meant," Sue recalls. She speaks in a monotone. "I went home and spent the night holding Marc and hugging Jesse. When the doctor called, he told me what I'd already guessed—the cancer had metastasized to my brain."

There is a pause in the story. When it spreads, breast cancer is most likely to travel to the lungs, the liver or the bones. In only about ten percent of all cases of metastases does it go to the brain.

Sue's eyes move around the kitchen past the antique wooden icebox she refinished and the white Formica cabinets she and Marc built together. She gazes out the greenhouse window at a white birch they planted years ago, but her mind turns inward to the future. "Why the brain? Why not the other breast? They could cut it off. Why not the bones? It's painful, but you could live a long time. But the brain? I don't want cancer in my brain. Now, my husband and I are planning for some difficult things. I gave Marc my power-of-attorney, and I've signed a living will and do-not-resuscitate orders. Marc barely knows the electric bill from the phone bill. Now we pay the bills together. And I always did our income tax. I'm showing him what to bring to an accountant next year."

Dealing with the details of everyday life gives Sue a way to cope. More than that, she wants to make sure people know she was here. She wants to be remembered.

"I'm in a hurry to finish a painting for Naomi. I'm working on a drawing for my parents. In the last trimester of my pregnancy, I had to stay off my feet, so I started embroidering a crib quilt. My daughter is almost three and it's still not done. I want to finish that stupid crib quilt. And I want to plant as many perennials as I can so that when I'm not here my flowers will brighten my family's days. Maybe they'll look at them and think of me and smile. I keep thinking will my little one remember anything about me?" And she lists some of the things she'd like Jesse to remember. "I love chicken. I could eat clams all day. I hate carrots. One summer when I was a kid, I played the violin. I love to dance."

Sue looks away from the window. "I know there are freak stories about people who were told they have two months to live, and they defy nature and live for years and years. Maybe I'll be one of those freaks. My husband tells me, 'You're going to make it Sue. You're going to live.' I look him in the eyes and say, 'You have to start facing reality, Marc.'"

Spring is turning into summer with a burst of purple foxgloves and the red and fuchsia impatiens Sue planted soon after Memorial Day. "I love feeling the earth," she said that morning from beneath the white floppy hat that shielded her from the sun. In the weeks since she planted the seedlings, Sue has hosted a third-birthday party for Jesse and a baby shower for Naomi. "I wish I could live long enough to see you have six girls who would put you through the kind of hell you put me through," she'd told her daughter as they opened presents. Naomi had laughed. "I'll just tell them, 'Go to Grandma's.'"

On a hot June day a week after the shower, Sue boards a Long Island Rail Road train for Manhattan, where she has a chemotherapy appointment with Dr. Greenspan. Her tote bag is crammed with a stack of unsigned petitions asking President Clinton to declare breast cancer a national epidemic and provide more funding for research. And she carries a bundle of envelopes for her bookkeeping clients that she wants Naomi to mail. When the train stops at a nearby town, Naomi is waiting on the platform. She takes the mail and hands Sue a rosebud.

"It's to let you know I'm thinking about you today," Naomi says, and she snaps an Instamatic photo of her mother before the doors close—a snapshot of a puffy-faced woman wearing a white canvas sun hat and black shorts and a T-shirt with a pink ribbon pinned over the heart as a symbol of breast cancer awareness.

It hasn't taken long for Sue Rosenbaum to become a breast cancer activist. Shortly after she was diagnosed, she joined "1 in 9," a grass-roots advocacy group, and became a member of its steering committee. In the spring of 1992, Sue marched in Washington. By summer, she was helping establish the Long Beach Breast Cancer Coalition, which would grow to 200 members and elect Sue Rosenbaum its first president. By January, she was spearheading an effort to document the cases of breast cancer in her community. Spring saw her back in Washington, and now, in the summer, the woman with tumors in her brain walks the Long Beach boardwalk when she's well enough, asking people to sign her petitions and fill out questionnaires for the local survey.

On the train, she keeps busy writing questions for Greenspan in a spiral notebook she carries to every medical appointment. Questions like "Can't put chin to chest, why? Stomach area tender for two weeks, why? Chemo not working? No more radiation? What else to do????" But as soon as she arrives at Penn Station, Sue Rosenbaum, breast cancer patient, becomes Sue Rosenbaum, breast cancer activist.

In the station, on subway platforms, on the E train and the No. 6, the bald woman in the white canvas sun hat smiles her big smile at strangers and holds out a clipboard with her petitions. "Too many women have breast cancer and I'm one of them," she says. Or "Something has to be done about breast cancer soon. Like yesterday." She says she'll take the petitions to Washington herself in the fall. Nobody refuses to sign.

By noon, Sue is in a treatment room in Greenspan's Fifth Avenue office. She wears a pink paper gown and sits on an examination table with a heating pad wrapped around her right forearm to bring out her veins. A nurse hooks up an IV of the anti-nausea drug Zofran.

Greenspan comes in—he's a short white-haired man with glasses and a limp who was once described by his famous patient comedienne Gilda Radner as having "a mashed potato face—a face you want to kiss. It was like going to see Mel Brooks or Willy Wonka for a medical opinion."

"What's doing?" he asks. "How are you feeling?"

"Look at me, I'm so swollen. I used to have bony ankles. Now, I have a triple chin and I move like an old woman." Then she zeroes in. "For weeks now, my entire body hurts—especially the whole chest area. When I cough or sneeze I have pain everywhere. If my little one drops something and I bend to pick it up, wow, woozy, I see stars. Why am I hurting so much, doctor?"

"I don't know. Cancer and chemotherapy will produce these aches and pains. Are the headaches getting better or worse?"

"Better than they were two, three weeks ago but worse than a few days ago. Doctor, is the chemo working? Why am I still getting these headaches?"

"Because you've got this damned condition, which is under partial control." A smile crinkles the mashed potato.

Sue remains stone-faced. "How long can I keep getting the chemo?"

"I had one patient who had chemo for five and a half years."

The nurse returns and administers a combination of chemo drugs that cause a burning sensation in her arm. "I'm burning," Sue yells. "I'm burning."

The nurse pats Sue's hand. "I'm sorry. Call me if it doesn't stop."

Sue shrugs. "I know the drill. It only lasts two or three minutes. Two or three minutes in hell." She takes deep breaths. She looks at the pink rosebud Naomi gave her. The nurse has put it in a vial of water.

While the chemo drugs drip into Sue's bloodstream, Greenspan sits in his paneled office lined with medical books and diplomas and citations, talking about his patient. A fax machine hums in the corner.

"Sue Rosenbaum has a cerebral metastasis," the doctor says. "This is very, very serious. Her cancer was of an infiltrating type, and there was a question as to whether the lungs were involved. The only way to handle it was with extensive chemo. Greenspan-style, meaning five drugs. With chemotherapy, it's not just a question of chemistry. It's chemistry and personality. Sue is a terrific patient. She never had a problem with tolerating the drugs. This girl has the most remarkable attitude. I know Sue is angry, but she seals her anger. She's angry because she figures she's only good for maybe another year or two, but that's looking for a miracle. I'm an optimist. I like to think that Sue's cancer is being arrested. The question is how long can we hold it back? No one knows. Her prognosis is not good. She's at an extremely high risk. The longest I've kept a patient like Sue going, the longest in my experience, is three and a half years. Whether I'll be that lucky with her I don't know."

Almost an hour later Sue's chemo session is over. "I'll give you ten days until the next time, but you have to have a blood count next Thursday—no later," Greenspan says. And he warns her about the possible side effects of the drugs. "If you develop mouth sores or black and blue spots anywhere on your body, call me immediately."

Sue looks frustrated. Greenspan goes on. "Now I want you to know, there's no patient in the United States like Sue Rosenbaum, and there's no doctor like Ezra Greenspan—we're a good team. You look terrific."

Sue clenches her jaw and narrows her eyes. "I feel like shit," she says.

Greenspan walks out of the room.

On her next visit, Sue waits in a tiny treatment room lined with shelves that are stuffed with patient files and alcohol swabs and syringes. When Greenspan enters, she bombards him with questions. "I feel tightness in my chest—should I have an EKG? What's causing the stiffness in my back? Why do I have pain in my legs—both legs, from my knees to my ankles?"

The doctor responds with a question of his own. "Do you have mouth sores?"

Sue shakes her head. She questions him about a new procedure called gamma-knife surgery in which hundreds of beams of radiation from thousands of angles come together to obliterate a brain tumor without the use of anesthesia or an incision.

"You have too many lesions."

Sue keeps at him. "What about this new drug for the brain you've mentioned?"

"It's supposed to penetrate the brain better, but it's experimental. I don't know yet if it's available or if it would be right for you."

"Well, when are you going to find out?"

Greenspan will make a call later to a colleague who is an expert on the new drug. He'll tell Sue it wouldn't be any more effective than the chemo he's already giving her. But for now he doesn't answer. He leaves the room.

Sue is feisty today. She expresses frustration her way. She gives her doctor the finger.

In early July, a time for blue hydrangeas and salmon-colored lilies, Sue and Marc drive to Memorial Sloan-Kettering for a consultation with Dr. Beryl McCormick, a radiation oncologist she has been referred to by Greenspan. Sue Rosenbaum's medical options are running out. She's searching for other ways to fight the malignancy closing in on her life. "If I could only get amnesia for a few days," she says.

Sue rests on an examination table in a blue hospital gown. Her face is still very puffy from steroids, and she hides under a floppy black hat with a sunflower pinned on the right side. Her paleness counterpoints Marc's tan. Her hands shake as she picks off her red nail polish.

Marc massages Sue's feet as they wait in the room with gray walls and a pastel curtain. He kisses her and tries to push away her sadness by talking about their honeymoon in the Poconos and a trip they took to Jamaica. At one point, Sue pulls her hat down over her face and curls up on the gray leather table.

She has herself under control when an associate of McCormick enters to ask her some questions. "I see that your last bone scans in February didn't show anything new. So right now it's just the tumor in your head you're worried about?"

"That's right. That's all."

Doctor and patient smile wanly.

"I see by your chart you have a three-year-old. You must feel tired a lot."

Sue chuckles. "Yeah. A three-year-old and breast cancer can really knock you out."

Dr. McCormick performs a neurological exam. Sue complains about weakness and leg pains. The doctor nods—both symptoms are side effects of Decadron, the steroid Sue is taking to improve penetration of the chemo drugs.

McCormick leaves to review the patient's records and brain scans, and Sue and Marc sit on the table holding onto hope and each other. When the doctor returns, she is very gentle and very serious. The effects of the radiation treatments Sue had received three months before should have been more lasting, she says. "There's evidence of progression on your scan. This is a very short interval. I'm really sorry, but I can't re-treat you."

Sue squeezes Marc's hand as McCormick continues: "Typically, you give a lesser dosage the second time around, but still there's an accumulation, and that can cause problems. If I were to give you a second round of radiation, it would have less of a response. It just isn't worth the risk, especially with multiple areas in the brain. I'd continue with chemotherapy and the Decadron and see what subsequent MRIs show. Right now you have one very large area."

"How large?" Sue interrupts.

"With the edema, probably eight to ten centimeters. Your biggest tumor is here." McCormick touches the sunflower. "The other lesions are smaller."

"How many other lesions are there?"

"It's hard to say how many. Many."

"Where are they?"

The doctor places her hand across the back of Sue's head.

Tears stream down Sue's face. "It's just that I want to know what's going on," she says. "It's hard to find somebody who will answer my questions."

"If the chemo keeps the lesions from progressing, if we can just see some stabilization in that larger area in the next six months, we can reconsider. Let's wait until the end of the calendar year and see where you are."

"So radiation is out," Sue says and she starts to cry. "I'm sorry," she tells the doctor.

Beryl McCormick reaches for Sue's hand, one human being touching another. "It's not easy for me to say we can't treat you. I want to treat you, but it would not be the wise thing to do right now. If you're stable, I'd be happy to see you at the end of the year. I'd really love to see you at the end of the year."

The woman who loves to dance moves slowly off the table. "I'm going to die, Marc," Sue whispers. "If the chemo doesn't work, I have no more options. I'm going to die."

"I'm not going to let you die. I love you too much."

Sue rests her head on her husband's shoulder. "How do I say good-bye to Jesse?"

It's August, and the pink hibiscus is in full bloom. Sue Rosenbaum is on her way to see her first grandchild. Her daughter Naomi lives with Minas Kinalis, the baby's father, but they are not yet married. When Naomi told her mother "you're going to be a grandma," Sue's reaction was pure Sue—direct but not judgmental. "I hope you know what you're doing," she said. Almost in the same instant, she hugged her daughter. "I love you, baby."

It wasn't always that easy. Naomi was ten when her parents divorced. "I resented my mom for sending my daddy away," she says. A year later she went to live with her father, who had remarried. "I knew she was upset, but I guess she was smart. She knew if she kept me from going, I'd resent her even more. When it came time to say good-bye, we were both crying. That's the way it always was with me and Mommy—we could never say good-bye without a lot of tears."

When she was thirteen, Naomi came home to her mother. They were fine until she started high school. "I wasn't a good student. I was never into drugs. I was just into myself and my friends. I barely graduated and then I moved out. But Mommy always left the door open. She helped me get an apartment, and she even stocked the refrigerator. A couple of months later I took off to join a boyfriend in Florida. Mommy couldn't believe it. She said, 'How are you going to manage without me?' I was there only a few weeks when I had to have my appendix out. I was scared, so I called Mommy from the hospital. She was there when I woke up—sitting by my bed, holding my hand."

That was in January 1989. Six months later Naomi returned to Long Island, and the mother and daughter rebuilt their relationship. The relationship remained unshaken when Naomi announced her pregnancy. Several months after that, in the living room of the house in Long Beach—Sue sitting in the mauve leather chair and Naomi on the plush charcoal-colored couch—they shared another wrenching moment. Sue's voice was flat. "I've always wondered, Naomi—did you get pregnant so I'd be alive to see my first grandchild born?"

She had to repeat the question before her daughter answered.

"When I first found out I was pregnant I was shocked. It wasn't like it was planned. I made a list of reasons why I should keep the baby and a list of reasons why I shouldn't. I wanted you to know my baby, Mommy. You were the number one reason on my 'should' list."

Sue's granddaughter, Alexis, was born on July 30 at 2:30 p.m. She weighed seven pounds, nine ounces. Sue visited the hospital, but only mothers and fathers were allowed to hold the newborns. She had to wait.

Now on this afternoon in August of 1993, Sue drives to her daughter's apartment, stopping off at Caldor's to buy nursing bras. She had a sleepless night thanks to a double dosage of steroids to alleviate another violent headache. And she's worried because her blood counts have been so low for the past three weeks that she hasn't been able to get chemo.

But her hair is growing because she hasn't been taking the drugs. She pulls off her white turban and rubs her head. It's a very uncharacteristic thing for her to do—she doesn't like to be seen without a hat or a scarf or a wig, especially around Jesse. A dark wisp curls at the nape of her neck and a streak of white runs down the middle of her head where the hair is thinner and her scalp shows. "I call this hairdo my reverse Mohawk with a sumo-wrestler tail."

Jesse giggles from the backseat. "Mommy, where's your head?"

Sue glances at her in the rear-view mirror. "I worry about all my girls. I pray none of them gets breast cancer. I know my granddaughter won't remember me, but I hope Jesse does a little bit. The day Naomi and the baby were discharged, Minas admitted his mother into the same hospital. She has lung cancer, and she's going fast. Poor baby Alexis isn't going to know either of her grand-mothers. I figure I might have at least another year. I know I'm getting worse, though. I see it in the mirror. Everything hurts."

But it's a day to smile through pain. "I'm going to hold my beautiful grand-daughter today. I'm on cloud nine."

Naomi is sitting on a blue couch in a living room where two parakeets sing in a cage and a black dog named Sheba chews a rubber ball. The television is tuned to "Oprah." A pink vase decorated with a yellow-haired baby sits on the TV. Sue got the vase as a present when Naomi was born and has given it to her daughter as an heirloom. A seascape dominates the room—the oil painting Sue was so anxious to finish for Naomi's twenty-third birthday.

Alexis is asleep in a white cradle. Jesse does her tiptoe dance around the room.

"I have to say hi to the baby," she announces and pirouettes over. "Hi baby Alexis." She stumbles against the cradle.

"Don't knock her over Jess," Sue yells even though the baby is undisturbed.

"She was very cranky last night," Naomi says. "I hardly slept."

Sue picks up her granddaughter. "Come here you."

She sits back on the couch with the baby on her lap. She kisses Alexis' cheek. "Hello, beautiful baby. I love you."

Alexis squiggles in her grandmother's arms and scrunches up her face.

Jesse inches closer. "Mommy, baby Alexis stuck her tongue out at you."

"Hey, gorgeous," Sue coos. "You have more hair than your nanny."

Roses and chrysanthemums sing a September song. The past few weeks have been cruel. Sue's headaches have become more maddening; her leg pains have worsened to the point where she's partially bedridden. She decided she couldn't make it into Manhattan anymore and found a doctor in nearby Rockville Centre. She hired an aide. Her blood counts dropped drastically, and she was hos-pitalized for transfusions.

Before she was admitted, she gave a friend her petitions for the president and the hand-made pink-and-black banner that the Long Beach coalition carries into battle. Her friend Mary Lou Monahan promised her that the banner would be carried past the White House.

The day before she went to the hospital, Sue stared at her bedroom wall and tried to exercise some control over death. "I want to die in my own bed with my family here at my side," she told her husband and a visiting nurse. "Please let me die at home." She pulled Jesse close. "One day, Mommy's going to go live with the angels."

Sue came home on September 14—her seventh wedding anniversary. She came home in an ambulance with Marc at her side. The place that has been his ever since he stood with her in front of a rabbi and stepped on a glass for luck.

Marc Rosenbaum had always been crazy about his wife. "When I first started seeing Sue," he says, "all my friends were like, 'Are you nuts? She's older, she's got a kid.' But none of that bothered me. She had great legs. She made a fantastic white clam sauce. She was the girl of my dreams.

"I loved to surf and Sue loved to ski. We loved to dance. But basically we were homebodies. I'd watch the hockey game downstairs and during intermission, I'd run up and hug her. We'd cuddle on the couch after Jesse went to bed. She made me a better person than I was. Sue taught me how to be a good father."

When she came home from the hospital, Marc told her, "Happy anniversary, Babe. Thank you for marrying me." But Sue didn't respond. He wasn't even sure she knew him.

Two days later, it was Rosh Hashanah, the Jewish New Year, and Marc returned from services facing reality. "I know she's going to die," he said, "but why does she have to be tortured? I broke down in temple when the rabbi talks about the Book of Life, about who will live and who will die in the coming year. I sat there and cried because I know my wife will die."

In late September Sue is confined to a hospital bed in her room. She is on morphine and gets a low dosage of steroid to reduce the swelling in her brain. Chemo has been discontinued. Three aides provide almost round-the-clock care, and the nurse, Kate Tormey, comes by every other day. Marc's mother, Rachel, and sister, Renie, are right next door. Sue's parents visit often. So does her sister, Carol Grogan, and her ex-sister-in-law Barbara Park.

On a Friday morning, alone in the house with his wife and daughter, Marc worries about Jesse's Halloween costume. It's the kind of thing Sue would have had all planned by now. Two years before Marc bought a chicken outfit that Sue transformed into a trophy winner at the Long Beach Halloween Parade. She designed a cracked eggshell out of oaktag and positioned it around a one-year-old Jesse so she looked like a baby chick who had just hatched. The next year Sue dressed up her little girl like a Chinese rickshaw driver, complete with a painted cardboard rickshaw—another award winner.

"Jess, how about being a daisy this year?" Marc asks.

Jesse makes a face and plays with her Cheerios.

"Eat your cereal nice, Jess Leigh. How about a ghost?"

"The little things in the Cheerios are gonna hurt me, Daddy."

"You always eat that cereal, you like that cereal. I know—you could be a princess."

"But what are those little things?"

"They're just bubbles in your milk, Jess. They won't hurt you."

"But they will. They'll float up into my head and give me a headache like Mommy has."

Marc kisses the top of his daughter's head. "No, baby, they won't. Would I give you something that would hurt you?"

He scoops up the Cheerios with her Little Mermaid spoon. "Do I have to feed you like you were baby Alexis?"

A few minutes later, Marc rummages through her dresser drawers. "Where's your watermelon shirt, Jess?"

"Mommy must have done something with it."

He washes her hands in the bathroom sink and watches her brush her teeth. He combs her brown shoulder-length hair that curls at the ends.

"Ouch," she screams.

"Come on. Please, Jessica. Your bus will be here any minute."

"But you're not doing it right. It never hurts when Mommy brushes my hair."

Jesse runs into the kitchen. Marc leans his head against the wall. "Oh, Sue," he cries, "please don't leave me. I need you."

Jesse tiptoes into her mother's room. "Morning Mommy," she calls.

Sue waves from her bed. "It's Jesse Bessie, my beautiful ballerina. Hi, big girl. Are you going to school today, gorgeous?"

Marc is composed when he enters Sue's room. He lowers the guard rail on the hospital bed so a little girl can crawl up and kiss her mother. Jesse throws her arms around Sue's neck.

"Oww." Sue winces and turns away.

Jesse runs out of the room. She goes into her bedroom and plays with Mr. Potato Head. Marc takes out the garbage.

The bus for preschool pulls up in front of the house. "I can go by myself, Dad."

Marc takes Jesse by the hand. "You have raisins in your bag for later," he tells her as he walks her onto the empty yellow bus. He smoothes back her hair.

"Jesse, what's this stuff all over your face? Oh my God, we forgot to wash your face. Jess, we gotta get the crud out of your eyes."

He jumps off the bus. "Back in a sec," he yells to the driver and reappears almost instantly with a wet washcloth. He scrubs Jesse's face. "Now you can go to school," he says and waves as the bus carries her away.

Back in the house, Marc talks to Druesilla Nesbitt, the aide who comes every day at eight in the morning and stays till four in the afternoon. "She was screaming all night," Marc says. "I don't know how much longer she can hold on."

"Yesterday was a grand day," Druesilla tells him. "I got her to sit on the commode chair for the first time. She held my hand and pretended to dance. She was laughing and singing, 'du-wa-ditty-ditty-dum-ditty-do.' She looked at me with those sad eyes and said, 'Why did this happen to me?' I had to look away so she wouldn't see me cry."

Marc folds up the studio couch in the living room, where he sleeps now that Sue is bedridden. Before he leaves for work, he looks in on his wife. Sue is dozing. She has dark circles under her eyes and sores on her nose and neck. Her mouth is open. Her hands shake. She's kicked off the covers.

Marc pulls a blanket over her. He caresses her cheek, and Sue opens her eyes.

"Is that Jesse crying?" she asks. "I can hear her. Why's she crying?"

"Jesse's at school, Hon."

Sue looks startled. She points to a corner of the ceiling. "Is the light darker over there?"

Marc bends over the railing and kisses her forehead.

"Watch it," she says. She laughs. "Kiss me again."

Marc kisses her on the lips this time. "Have a good day, Babe."

"Yeah, I think I'll go shopping."

They both laugh. "I love you," they say simultaneously.

Sue drifts back to sleep. Dru sits in a chair by her bedside. The room is warm and dark and quiet. Sue rubs her eyes. She chews her fingers. Suddenly she wakes up.

"Baby Alexis is dead," she says. "They're not telling me, but I know." She looks frightened. "I have dreams about it."

She throws off the blanket and grabs the chrome guard rail. "When am I going to die?" she whispers.

As fall deepens and the impatiens cling to life in the garden, the cancer continues to scar Sue's body and eat at her soul. She barely talks for days, her periods of lucidity become fewer and fewer. "I have tarantulas on my head," she says. "Ssshhh, don't tell anyone."

One evening, Jesse stops the visiting nurse. "How come my mommy wears a diaper?" And then Jesse repeats what her mother told her while she was being potty-trained. "Big girls don't wear diapers."

The nurse, Kate Tormey, pulls Marc aside. "Her death is imminent."

Marc sighs. "I was hugging her earlier tonight, telling her, 'I love you, Sue.' She hasn't spoken in days, but she opened her eyes and said, 'This is a bunch of crap.' Boy is she right. When the person you know isn't the one who's in there anymore, it's very hard. I wish she could just jump out of bed and be Sue again."

He spends the next few hours on the couch—holding Jesse in his lap and looking at photo albums and videos. On screen, Sue escorts a chubby toddler on a walk through the garden in the backyard. "Come on you gorgeous girl. Come see Mommy's flowers." Sue's voice is clear and strong and happy. She picks a pink flower and puts it behind Jesse's ear.

Sue is in Florida, holding her daughter's hand and feeding Cheerios and cheese doodles to ducks. Sue does a great duck imitation until one nips at Jesse's fingers. Sue snatches her away from harm and kisses her. "Bad duck." Sue walks off camera, but her voice keeps going. "Oh, did he scare you?"

In the darkened living room Jesse calls out, "Don't go away, Mommy."

Marc turns to a picture in their wedding album. Sue holds a champagne glass. She's smiling her big smile. "To you, Babe," Marc says. He touches her face.

60

"Look at that face. No one will ever love me like she did. Who else is going to tolerate my singing?"

He pulls Jesse close. "I know I have to find a way to show my daughter that the world is still beautiful, that the flowers come back in the spring and the waves keep crashing on the shore. But how?"

Then he goes into Sue's room, where he lowers the guard rail and leans to whisper good-bye.

Minutes later, Naomi stands at the bedside. She rubs her mother's cheek. "You don't have to hold on anymore, Mommy," she says. "You can go where it's peaceful. It's okay. You can rest now."

Day by day over the next week, Sue Rosenbaum fades like a flower in fall. She dies on October 25, a little before seven in the morning. She is forty-two years old.

There are two farewells for Sue Rosenbaum—a service in a funeral home where a rabbi reads the eulogy written by her family and friends and the gathering in the garden.

And then a month later, two days before Thanksgiving, when darkness silhouettes the dogwood and the crab apple trees, Marc walks across the street to the esplanade. Naomi follows with baby Alexis bundled in her arms. Jesse is with her sitter.

Marc looks up at the pale stars in the somber sky. Then he kneels to touch the hard brown earth. He sprinkles his wife's ashes in the garden she planted and nurtured, where crimson chrysanthemums hold on and a few pink roses live beyond their time.

He thinks about the seasons to come. "Make the flowers grow, my love," he says.

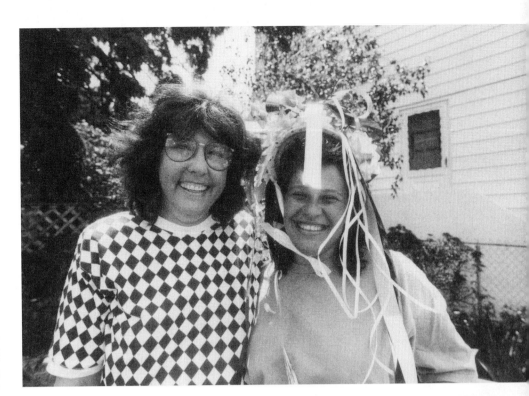

A wedding shower
Sue Rosenbaum makes it
to the shower for her
daughter Naomi, clearing
another hurdle.

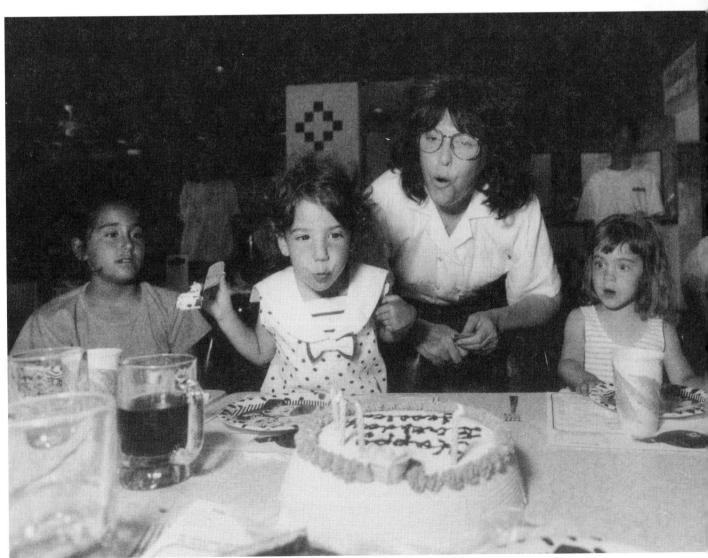

Still a mom, too
Jesse blows out the candles at her third birthday party, featuring a cake made by Mom.

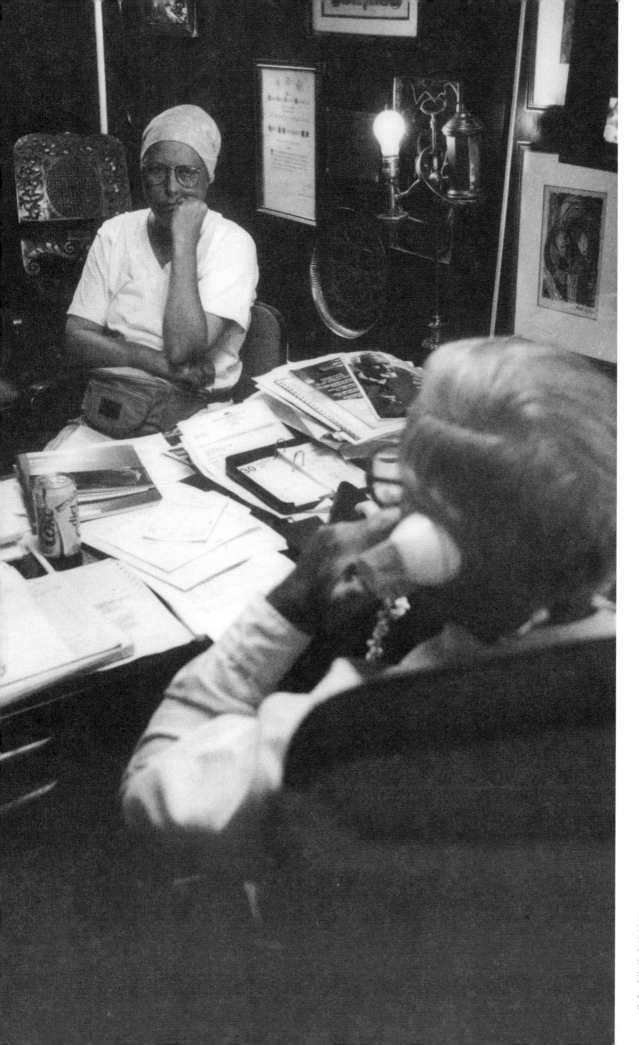

It's the waiting
Sue Rosenbaum waits
for her oncologist, Dr.
Greenspan, to get off
the phone and answer
some of her questions.
Waiting for answers is
one of the more frus-
trating parts of the day.

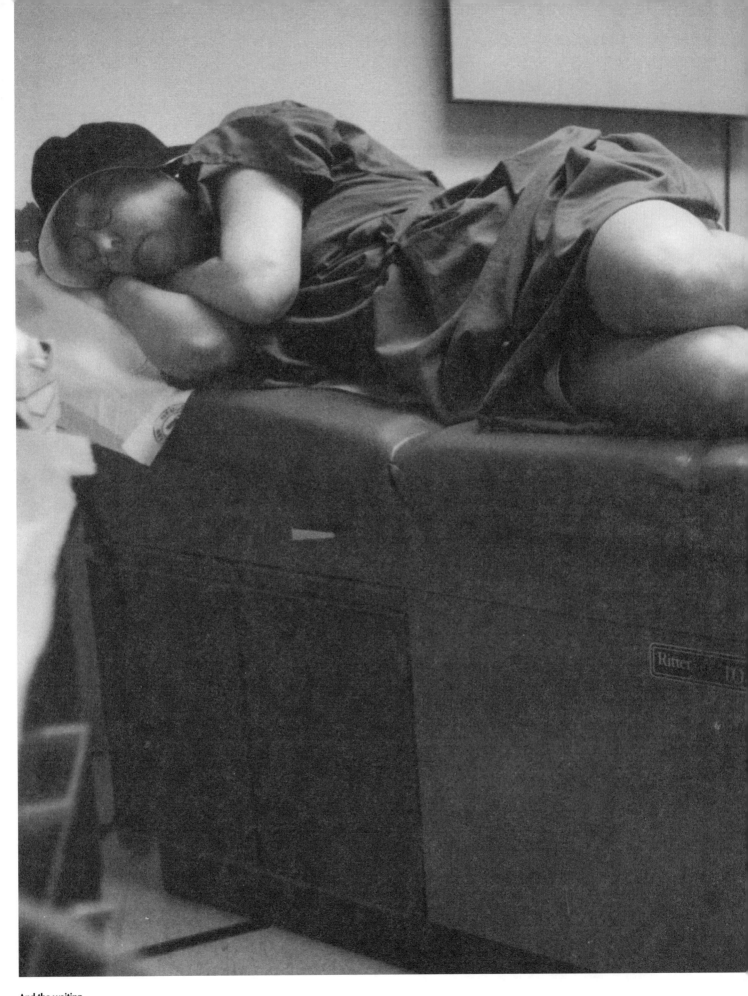

And the waiting. . .
Sue and Marc Rosenbaum wait for the radiologist to tell them whether she is well enough for additional treatment, a wait that ends in the agony of being told there's nothing more to be do

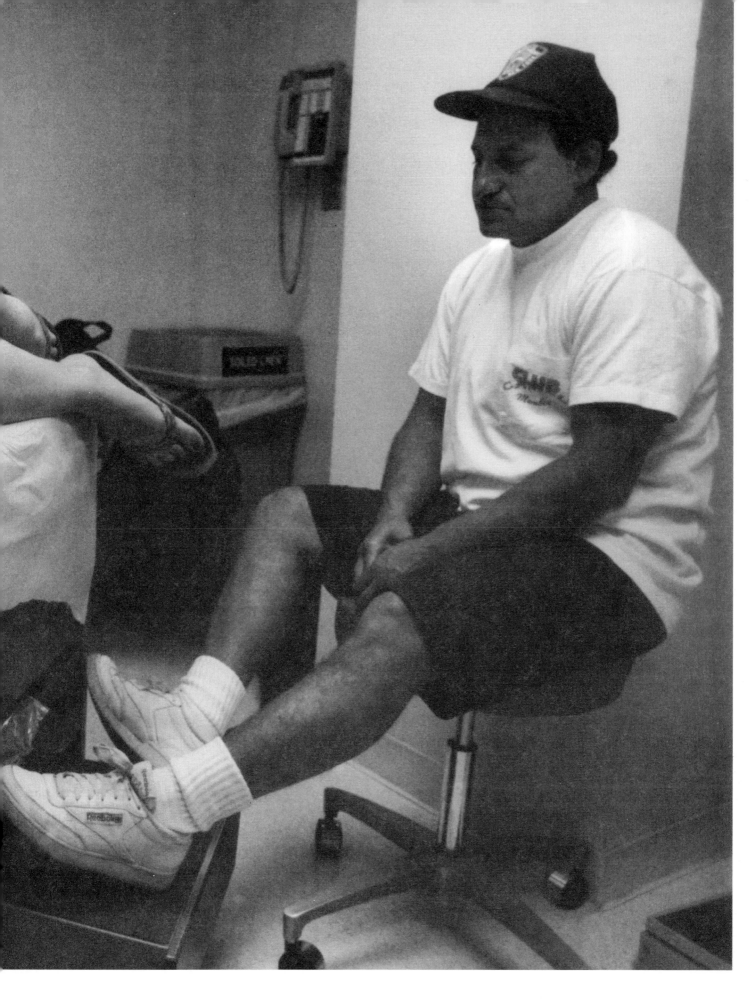

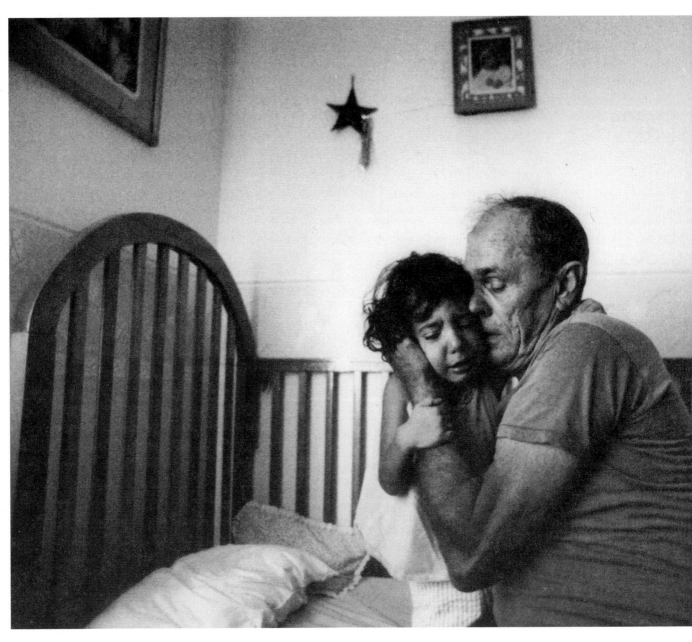

Where's Mommy?
Jesse wakes up from a nap crying for her mother, who is napping in the next room, and she needs the comforting words of grandpa Bill Lord, Sue's father.

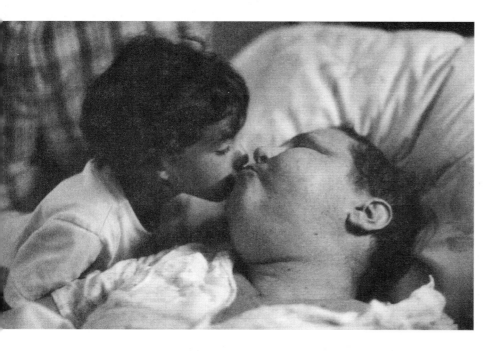

Kiss for Mom
Jesse remembers to kiss her mother before going out. Sue has a few weeks to live.

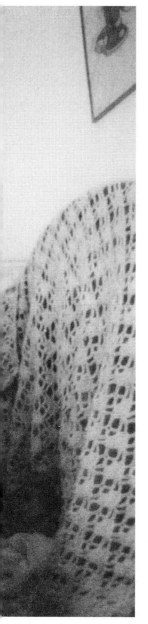

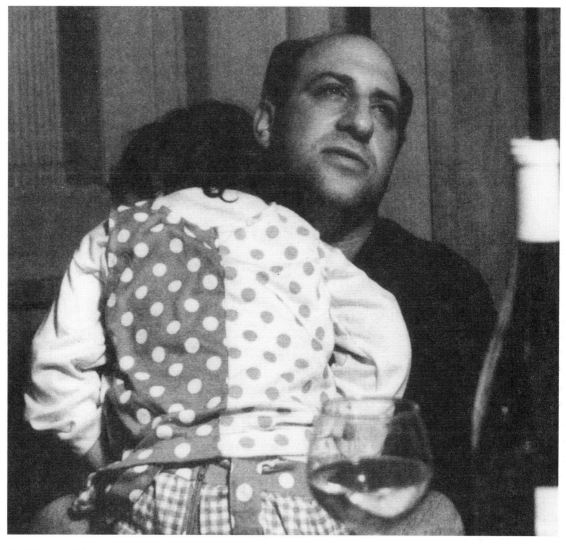

What do you say?
How do you tell a little girl that her mother might not live through the night? Marc Rosenbaum just holds Jesse and sits quietly.

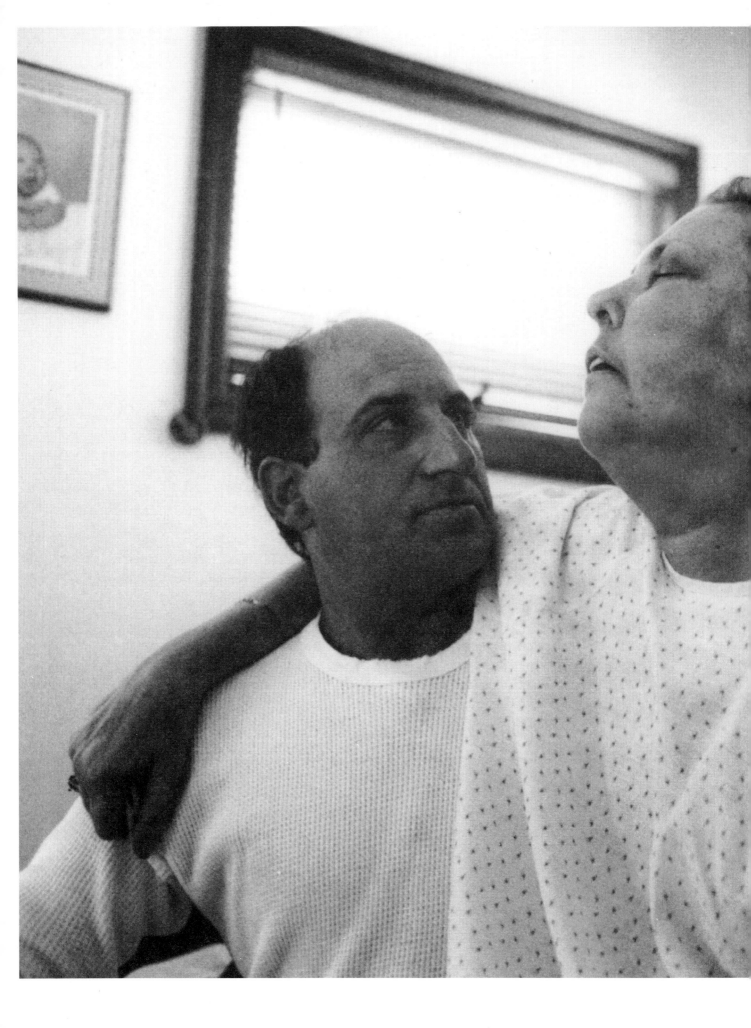

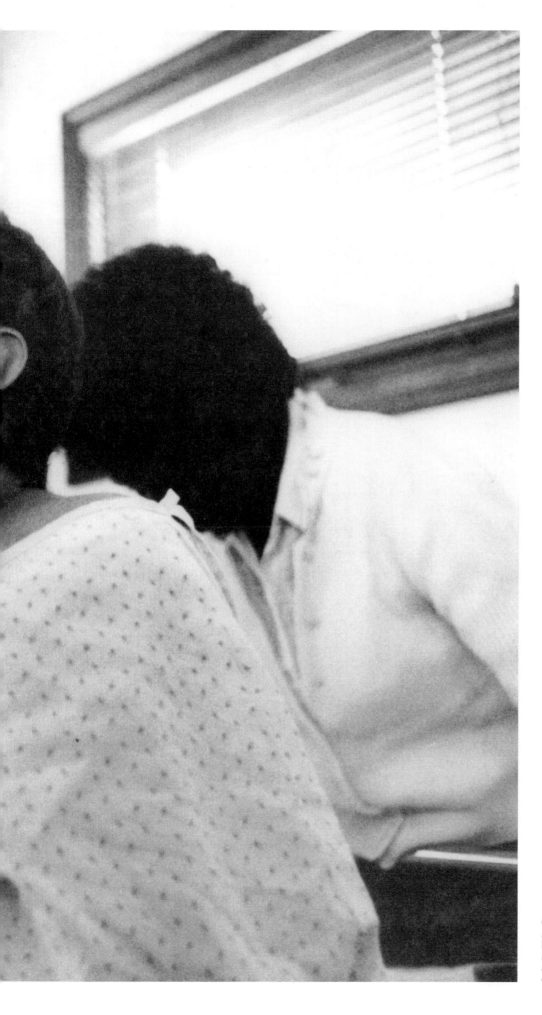

Changing sheets
As moving around
becomes more painful,
Marc holds Sue while
a visiting nurse
changes the sheets.

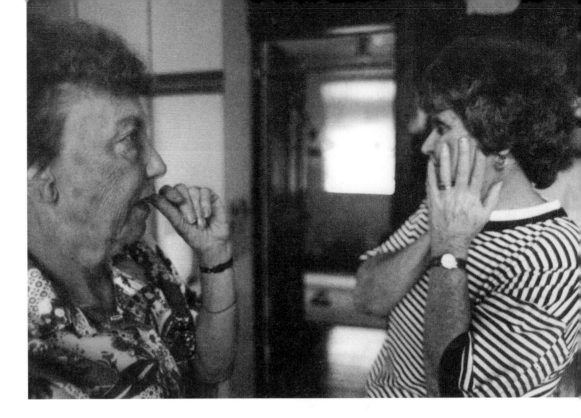

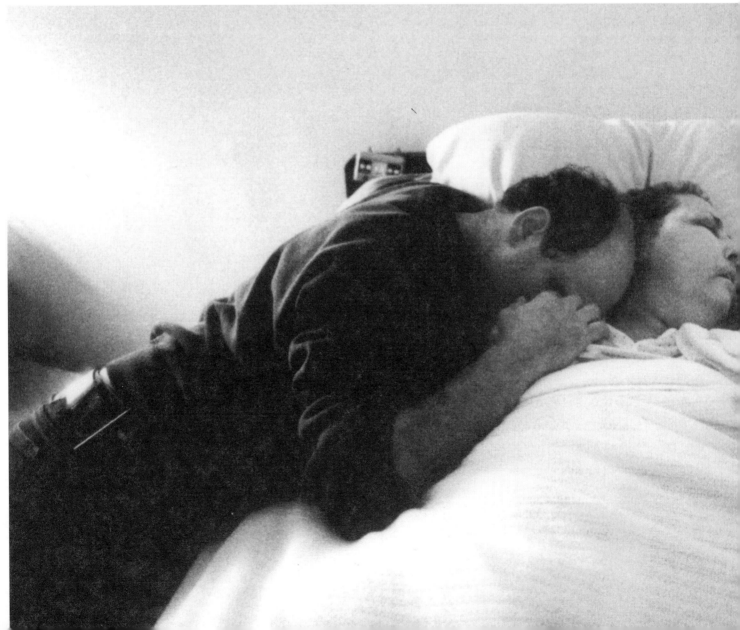

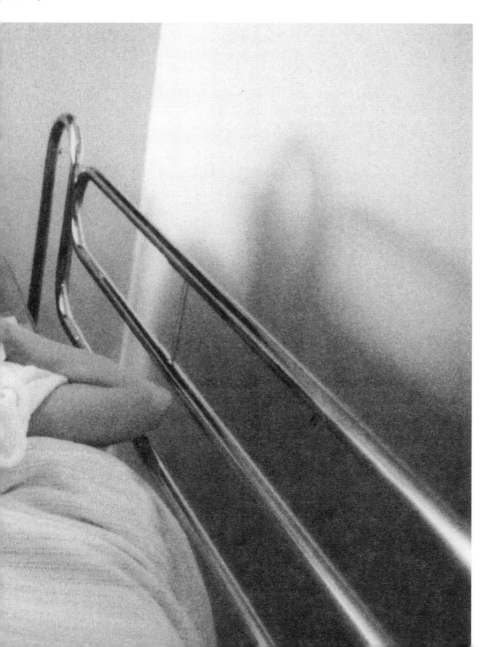

t this
's mother, Irene Lord,
 neighbor Terry
Connor learn of her
 eless condition
 know it's simply a
tter of days.

When to say good-bye
Marc learns that Sue,
falling in and out of
consciousness, is not
expected to live
through the night.

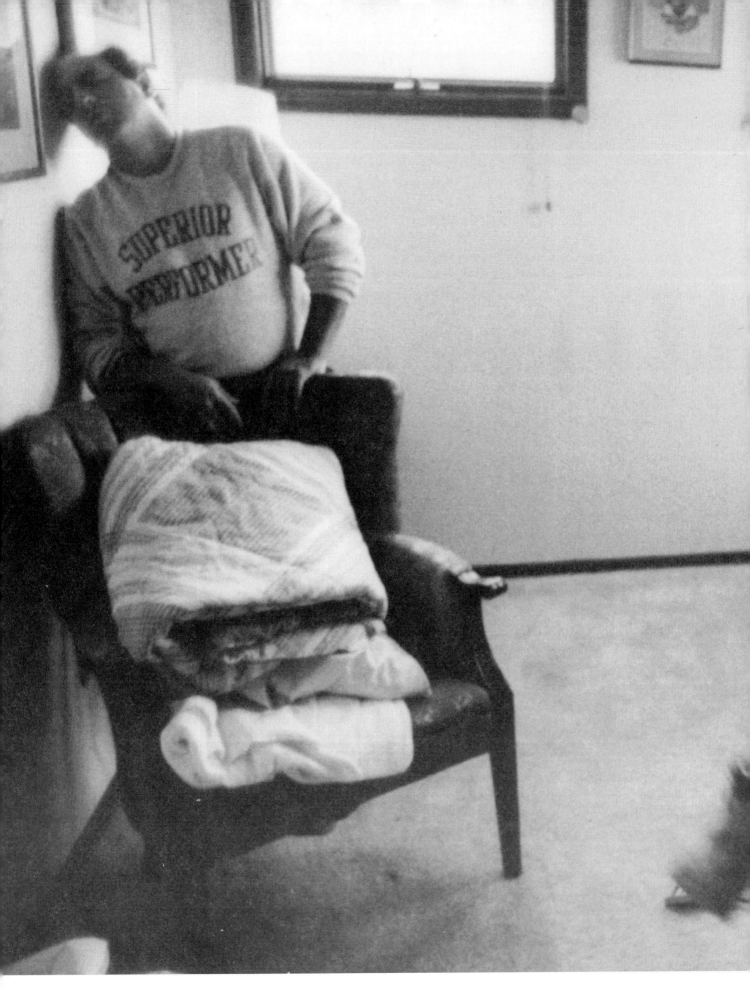

Mourning
Marc leans against the wall as a worker removes the hospital bed from his home.

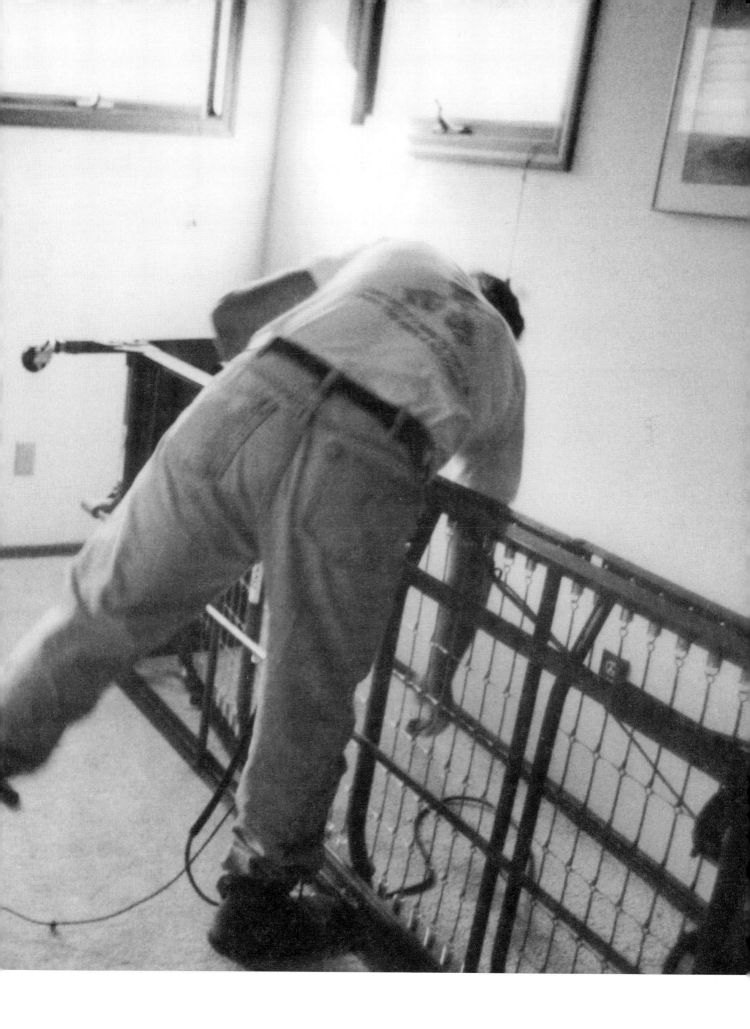

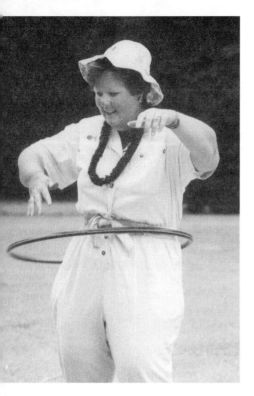

Party animal
Liz LoRusso hula-hoops it up at a block party.

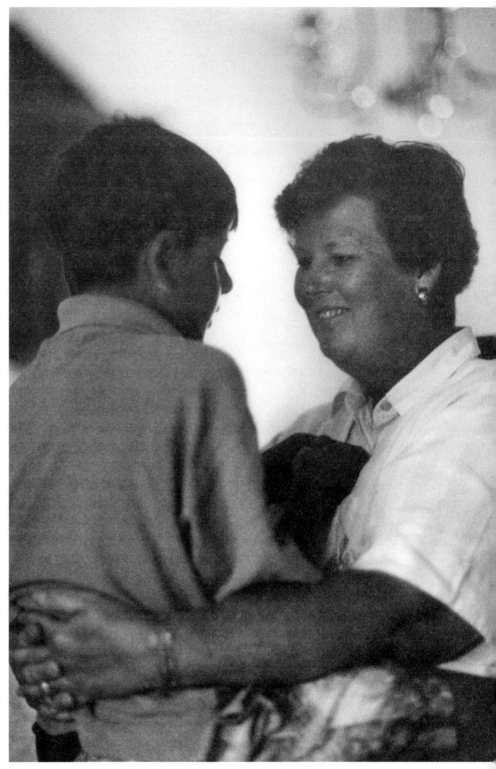

I'm still your mom
Liz LoRusso holds her son, Philip.

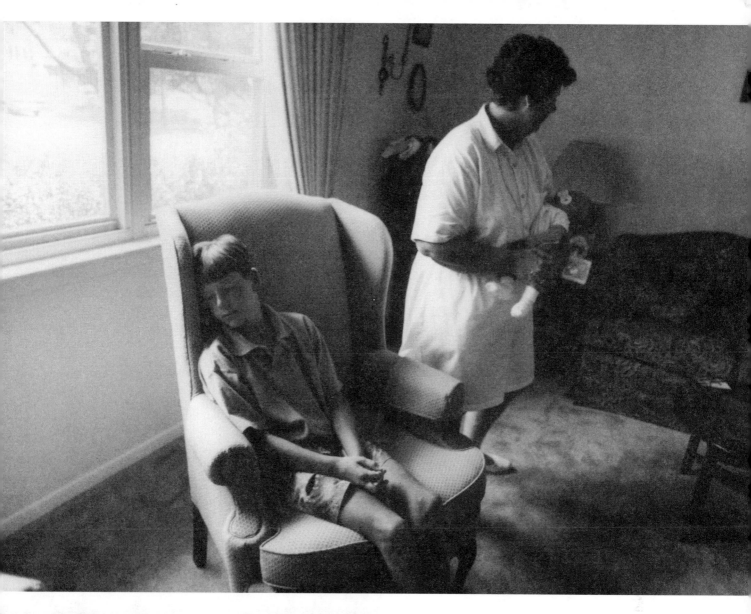

Too little time
Liz holds her new nephew while Philip looks away.
Even today, he rarely says the words "breast cancer."

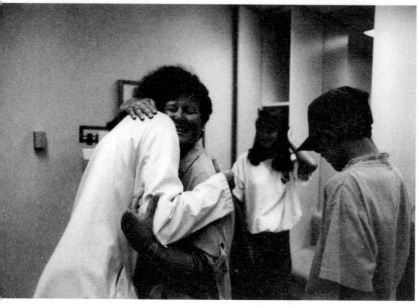

od news
hugs her doctor after a good
ckup while Philip and daughter
ren look on. Now they'll spend
afternoon enjoying Manhattan.

Another beach season passes
"I tell my kids what the
doctors tell me—I'm treatable
but not curable . . . I tell them
I love them; I love being their
mommy and I love being
alive. I know it will take a
miracle for me not to die of
this disease—but I believe
in miracles."

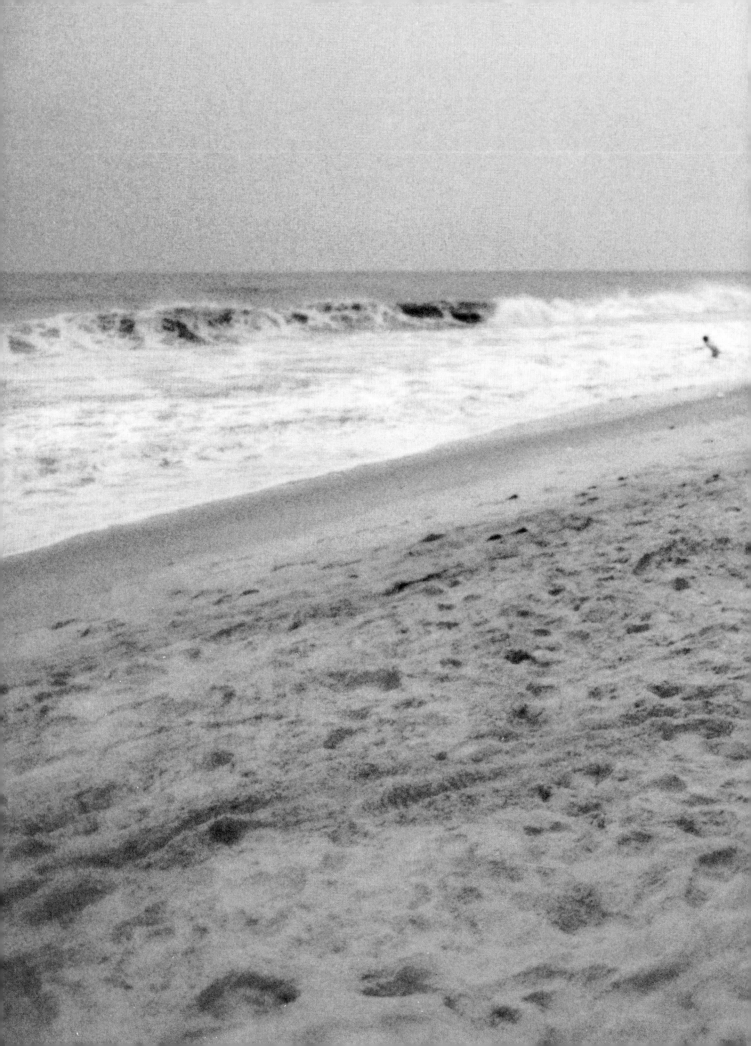

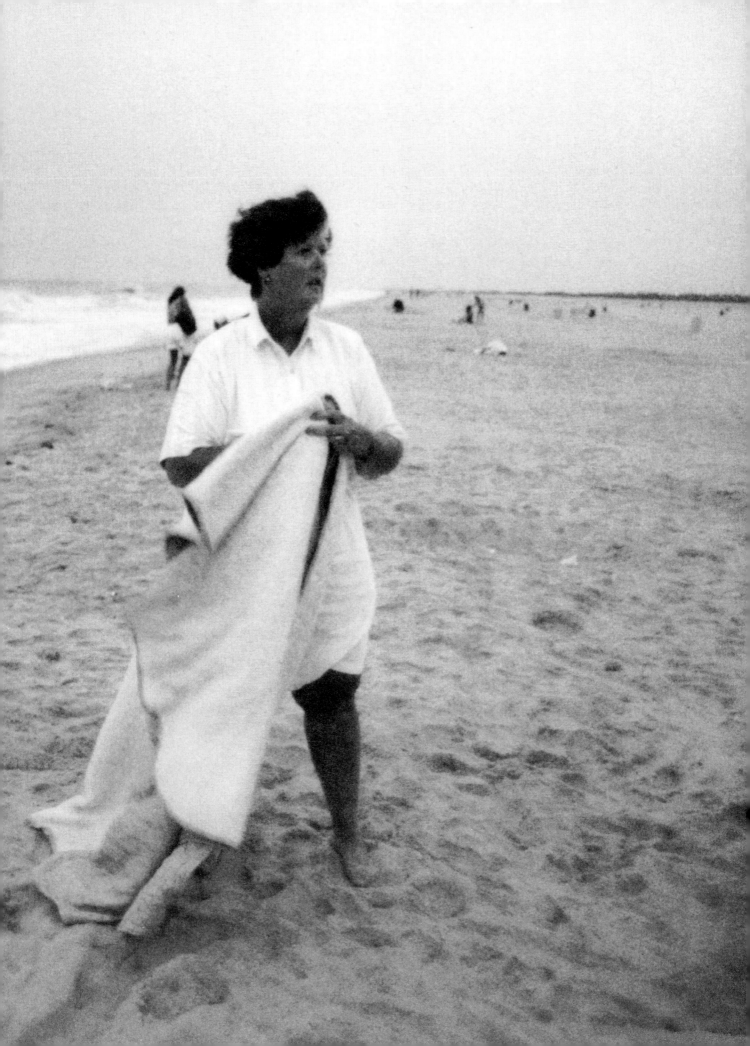

CHAPTER 6

—

Daphne Jackson: A Survivor

When Daphne Jackson felt a hard knot just below her right armpit almost three years ago, she made an appointment with her doctor but she didn't worry about breast cancer. The very idea seemed ridiculous.

A few days before the checkup, she sat alone in the back row at a seminar on breast cancer sponsored by her church. When a silicone breast with a suspicious lump was passed around, Daphne remembers feeling it and thinking, "Gee, it's hard—like mine." But that's as far as she went. She looked at the women in front of her—women in their fifties and sixties—and thought what she had always thought: Breast cancer is for older women. Not for her. She was only twenty-seven.

"Even the breast surgeon didn't seem worried and I felt like I was just being guided through the proper procedures to confirm that everything was okay," Daphne says. "When I had to have a sonogram because they said I was too young for a mammogram, I felt like, 'See, there's not even a question of breast cancer because I'm not an old woman.'"

The first glimmer came the day before the cancer was confirmed. She watched Magic Johnson talking on television about AIDS. She admired his courage and thought: "If I find out I have a life-threatening illness, I'll never make it through, I'll never survive."

When the doctor called at her job as a database administrator in Manhattan and told Daphne the worst, her boss arranged for a car and driver to take her home to Hempstead, on the western edge of Long Island.

"I sat in the back seat of a black Lincoln Town Car and all I could think was 'I'm going to die. I'm twenty-seven and I know what I'm going to die from.' I remember thinking, 'I should make out a will.' And my next thought was, 'But I haven't even started to live—I have nothing to leave to anyone.' I kept telling myself, 'I have to prepare for this. How do I prepare to die? Why me? I go to church—okay, maybe not every Sunday, but often. I live right, I eat right, I work hard, I'm nice to people—I've done nothing to be punished for.' That's how I looked at breast cancer—it was a punishment for something. And it was a death sentence.

"All the way home I kept thinking of the things I'll never be able to do. Get married, have kids, own a house. Travel—I've hardly been anywhere outside of New York. And now my future was being taken away from me. It was like tomorrow was my last day on earth."

When Daphne got home that day her father, James, was leaving for his job in a grocery store warehouse. He waited until his wife, Mable, arrived. Two-

and-a-half years later, at ease in the yellow kitchen of her parents' home where she lives, Daphne remembers the scene:

"My mother said, 'Why're you home, D?'"

Mable Jackson—a petite woman in a pink housedress and slippers—has been reading the newspaper at the table. Daphne turns to her. "Do you remember what I said, Mama?"

Mable pulls her glasses down on her nose and peers at her only daughter. "I didn't teach you to lie but you lied to me that day."

That day, Daphne told her mother: "I have cancer, Mama."

Mable Jackson couldn't believe it. She tore through the house, yelling, "Not my baby. It can't be. I'm supposed to go before you."

Daphne cries as she tells the story. Her mother keeps reading the newspaper. Without looking up, she hands her daughter a tissue. Daphne dabs her eyes and continues:

"She ran downstairs, upstairs, room to room, screaming. 'No, no, no. Take me; don't take my girl. Please let her live.' I said, 'Mom I need you to come with me to the doctor.'"

Mable Jackson's response stunned Daphne: "'No,' she said. 'I can't, I won't take you to no doctor because this is not true.'"

Now, Mable Jackson looks up from the newspaper and says quietly: "I didn't believe it then and I still don't believe it. Cancer doesn't run in this family—nowhere down the line, on either side. So how could she have it? It has to be something else, something that would have disappeared by itself. I'll never believe that my daughter has cancer and it bothers me that she believes it. Daphne shouldn't have had that operation."

Daphne remembers embracing her mother. "I put an arm around her and said, 'It'll be all right, we'll get through it.' My father took me to the doctor that day. He took the day off. The doctor was talking, going over my options, but I was in my own world. She asked if I had any questions. I couldn't think of any questions. I couldn't even hear. And my dad, he didn't know what to ask."

Daphne had a lumpectomy on December 11, 1991. Like most breast cancers, hers was detected in its early stage. Radiation treatments started about five weeks later, followed by six months of chemotherapy. Daphne continued working. "It was my way of pushing it all out of my mind. I wanted my life to be normal."

Normal during those months meant driving for treatment at Long Island Jewish Hospital, then driving to catch a train into the city to work. "I'd spend my lunch hour in the medical section of Barnes and Noble across the street. I'd read books on breast cancer on the train home, trying to learn what was happening inside my body, trying to understand a new language, trying not to think about what it all meant."

Her women friends and a support group at Adelphi University were Daphne's lifelines. "My mom and dad were in denial from the beginning. They wouldn't go to the doctor with me. My friend Audrey took me. My mom would say, 'I can't take you to the doctor because you don't have cancer.' She thinks it was a benign growth from the deodorant I was using or something like that. My dad wasn't feeling well and he'd say, 'I'm too tired.' They were so far into denial that to go with me they'd have had to admit that this is real."

When her chemo ended last July, Daphne started thinking about the tomorrows she once thought would be denied her. She took the training course to be a volunteer on the breast cancer hotline run by Adelphi. She remembered her own feeling of loneliness when she learned she had cancer.

"I was twenty-seven and there was no one around who was my age who was going through it," Daphne says. "Now, maybe I can be there for someone else who is young and frightened."

In January she quit her job with a publishing firm and enrolled full-time in a one-year certificate program in computer graphics and design—a step toward realizing her dream of starting her own computer consulting firm.

The only visible mark of Daphne Jackson's journey through breast cancer is a two-and-a-half-inch scar on her right breast. But her optimism hides other scars. Daphne lives with the ghost of cancer past—a ghost that is especially foreboding for a woman who is young and single. "It's difficult to tell someone I'm dating I've had breast cancer. I always stopped myself. I'll think, 'Wait awhile. Daphne, and see how things go before you spill your guts.' Breast cancer is the reason I'm not seeing anyone right now. I'm afraid of rejection. Who would want to be bothered with a twenty-nine-year-old woman who's had breast cancer? I'm not ready to deal with a man telling me he can't get involved because he's afraid I might die. I'm not ready for that."

Several months ago, Daphne met a man from Texas at a seminar in Manhattan and they started a friendship over the phone. "I was always telling him I did this or that related to breast cancer but he never asked why. He called one night when I was in a hurry to watch a breast cancer special on TV. This time he asked, 'Why are you so active in breast cancer? Did you ever have it?' I was scared but I wasn't going to lie. So I told him." She expects her friend to visit her this weekend.

"I want to get married and have kids and live the life I dreamed of," Daphne Jackson says, and then she thinks about the illness that makes no guarantees for the young. "And I don't know if I ever will. Sometimes I still cry over it."

DAPHNE JACKSON: *My friends would try to get me out of the house but every night, I'd read, read, read about breast cancer. It was like I was reading about someone else but I couldn't stop. And I couldn't cry—not a hard cry. I'd tear every now and then. But I couldn't cry for real—I was too busy trying to block it. Crying came a long time afterwards—a few months after chemo was over. I came home from my support group. I'd been talking a lot that night. I came home to clean up my room. There were all these books and magazines and pamphlets about cancer and chemo and radiation all over the place. Everything I'd been reading for months. I thought, "This is my life. How did this happen? This isn't right. Not for me. Not for a twenty-eight-year-old." And I sat down on the floor and I cried.*

Helen Meyrowitz: A Survivor

Almost one year after her mastectomy, Helen Meyrowitz went into mourning for her left breast.

It was an epiphany on a soft summer night in 1978. A sudden and overwhelming moment that would stretch into hours of sobbing for the woman Helen had been and could never be again.

A moment that comes to most breast cancer victims. A moment of visceral understanding that breast cancer had forever changed her life.

That day, Helen and her husband, Sid, had sunbathed on a beach in East Hampton. They were resting in the cabin of their thirty-one-foot motorboat anchored offshore when the day seized Helen Meyrowitz. Without warning, she started to cry.

Not just tears but sobs and sighs and hiccups and wails that shook her body through the night.

"What's wrong?" her husband asked. It was hours before she could stop crying long enough to answer.

Like a child, Helen Meyrowitz, a mother of two, finally sat up on the bunk and wiped her nose and eyes with the back of her hand. "I can never wear a bikini again," she whispered and started to cry again.

Sid reached for her. "But the surgery was a year ago," he said. "Besides, you're beautiful."

Helen continued to sob. She'd fought so hard since the mastectomy to swallow her fear, to feel in control. An artist, she'd stifled panic attacks with long sessions in the studio of her home in East Meadow, one of Long Island's early suburban developments, and long walks in her neighborhood. She'd told herself that losing her breast was nothing compared to losing her life.

66

But at that moment of mourning, the thought wasn't enough. It wasn't enough to counteract the day she'd spent on the beach in a high-neck one-piece suit and prosthesis watching other women romp around in bikinis. She was embarrassed by her own vanity, but she couldn't hold back the tears.

"It hit me that I wasn't who I'd always been. I was now a woman with only one breast. The breast is such a goddamn symbol. It's all wrapped up in how we see ourselves and how we think other people see us. I was ashamed to realize that I was capable of such vanity. I kept thinking, 'I'm still here, I'm alive—so why am I crying about a pound of fat?' And suddenly it was like a pressure cap had been removed. When you're looking at death, I think you must have a certain amount of denial. But after a while, you have to let yourself mourn your loss in order to move on."

Helen Meyrowitz moved on.

She made changes that have become the heart and soul of her days and years. Changes for the body, changes for the spirit. Changes she might never have dreamed of before the lump in her left breast was discovered in 1977. She was forty-eight years old then, her son and daughter were old enough to be on their own. She was an artist who'd completed her bachelor's degree in fine arts and showed her work in museums and galleries. She'd had a scare the year before, when she felt a lump that was aspirated. The lump was benign and the doctor told her to come back for six-month checkups.

At the one-year anniversary, the doctor found another lump in the same spot, and Helen Meyrowitz felt as if her body had betrayed her. "I'd always felt I could handle anything. But suddenly I was in a situation where I had no tools from any past experience to help me."

It was a time when breast cancer invariably meant a radical mastectomy— a deforming operation in which the pectoral muscles are removed in addition to the breast. A time when lumpectomies were unheard of, and modified radicals were a relatively new procedure. It was a time before breast cancer support groups. A time before chemotherapy was an almost-automatic prescription or breast cancer was a suitable topic for a TV talk show.

Helen Meyrowitz didn't know anyone who'd had breast cancer, but she knew that Happy Rockefeller, the wife of then-governor Nelson Rockefeller, had undergone a mastectomy a few years before. "When I suddenly had to find a surgeon, I went to Happy Rockefeller's doctor in Manhattan. His associate did my mastectomy. In those days, when you went for a biopsy, you had to sign a release for them to do a radical. I put myself in the hands of the doctor, who was God— that's the way it was. I didn't know to ask questions, and doctors didn't talk to you like they do now. I was fortunate because my doctor was on top of the latest developments and he did a modified radical. When I was awake and realized I was alive, I felt great relief. I didn't want to think beyond that."

Now every morning before breakfast, Helen and Sid, a retired furrier, walk two and a half miles in their neighborhood. In bad weather, Helen does thirty minutes on a stationary bike and works out with three-pound weights for twenty minutes. Then she does a half-hour of yoga. She spends most of her day painting in the high-ceilinged, glass-walled studio that was added onto the house she and Sid moved into as young-marrieds in 1952.

Life added new dimensions to art. Helen Meyrowitz the artist changed, too.

"My work is like looking in a mirror. It's my key to knowing myself. In the past, my figures were floating in a void or abstract space, sometimes tethered by umbilical cords or restraints, I never decided which. They were always gray and isolated and alienated, and the space around them was dark and frightening. Since the breast cancer, my work is very free and much more colorful. I returned to a series of falling figures, but now they're in a landscape. They're more energetic and vibrant. I think they're still saying that man is out of sync with nature and the environment—but now it's not as personal. There's more humor and understanding that it isn't easy to survive, that life is a struggle, but there is a light at the end of the tunnel—and it isn't just another train coming to run you over."

At five p.m., Helen meditates for twenty minutes, then starts dinner. Diet is one of the places where the changes are pronounced—starting with the elimination of red meat. "When you have cancer, you don't feel like you have control of anything," she says. "At first that sense of control comes from holding on for dear life. But then I saw that in order to truly gain control again, I had to see if I could let go. Let go of assumptions about my life and my self. Diet was an easy and obvious place to start."

Helen's diet is low-fat and mostly vegetarian, with a little fish and poultry thrown in. Grains, pasta, fresh fruits and vegetables—organically grown when she can find them. She takes vitamin supplements and uses a juicer. She and Sid don't consume caffeine or refined sugar, and Helen is pleased that her four-year-old granddaughter is being raised without meat or sugar. "I loved cake and ice cream. Now I don't even like the taste of sweets."

From the beginning, she had her husband's support. "After the operation I was afraid there'd be no physical attraction," Sid says. "I remember thinking, 'What does a guy do when this happens to his wife?' The surgery was in February, and in the spring we went to the Virgin Islands. That was a turning point for me—the realization that my feeling had more to do with the total woman. It was a marvelous revelation that my love wasn't based on an outer shell, a body, a breast. I realized my wife is part of myself and I had to change along with her."

Helen had started walking, and one Sunday Sid said he'd join her. To his surprise, he couldn't keep up. "I went out for three weeks by myself; then I said, 'I'll go with you again.' We walked together every day and slowly we started jogging. When we jogged our first mile, it was like we'd climbed Mount Everest. We ran two miles a day for ten years. Now we do fast walking. We were doing a twelve-minute mile when we jogged. We do a thirteen-and-a-half-minute mile when we walk."

Sid Meyrowitz remembers the day his wife cried for her lost breast. "It was hard for me because of her feelings about herself," he says. "I didn't want her to feel less of a woman because she couldn't wear a bikini. I love her."

Seventeen years after her mastectomy, Helen gets regular checkups and mammograms, but both she and Sid feel that cancer is behind her. "To me, a recurrence is as remote a possibility as my house exploding. Now and forever my mission is to live day by day and live each day as fully as I can."

Her mourning is long over. Helen Meyrowitz is happy about the woman she has become. "I learned that I'm not as fragile as I thought I was," she says. "And I learned that my mind is the most important part of my anatomy. I don't advocate breast cancer as a way to change—but if that's the challenge you're facing, I'm here to say you can grow from it in some unexpected and very positive ways."

HELEN MEYROWITZ: One day—it was in November of 1976—I looked at my bra on the bed and as an artist I thought, there's something interesting here. It was a satin underwire bra and I found it fascinating—the way it would collapse when I took it off and threw it on the bed. It inspired me to start a series of drawings that was highly unusual for me. I'd always drawn figures so why would I suddenly start drawing my own clothing? My shirts, my bikini, my bras. Mostly my bras, hanging empty without breasts or bodies in them. My art is a road map of my psyche and even though I wasn't aware of it at the time, something was going on inside me. Maybe it was a premonition or a preparation for something to come. Maybe it was my unconscious fear, having had a benign lump aspirated nine months before. But to me, that series of empty bras was an amazing phenomenon. Two months after I watched in fascination as my satin underwire bra collapsed on the bed I was told I had to have a mastectomy.

Thomasine Dembo: A Survivor

Georgia Montague and Thomasine Dembo were more like sisters than mother and daughter—they both had high cheekbones and ready smiles and a gift for easy conversation. They took trips together and went shopping together, they even lived next door to each other. So when Georgia Montague felt something strange in her breast she turned to her only daughter.

They were floating in the above-ground pool in Georgia's backyard one afternoon and more than twenty years later Thomasine still remembers her mother's words. "Tommy, I don't like the way my breast feels. Come, I want you to feel it."

It was as if her mother's right breast had turned to stone. "It was hard as a rock," Thomasine says, "especially around the nipple." She said, it didn't hurt. It took some doing, but I finally convinced her to see a doctor."

Georgia Montague had a radical mastectomy in 1975 and the daughter suffered through the mother's breast cancer almost as if it were her own. "She faced it better than I did. Like it was any other operation. She said, 'Tommy I've lost my breast.' I didn't want her to see the weakness in me but I couldn't help it—I cried like a baby. She didn't. She said, 'Hush now. It's over and done with.' She was happy-go-lucky right away. That was my mother—she never worried about nothing."

But within one year the stately fifty-two-year-old woman from North Carolina who worked as a seamstress and who raised two sons and a daughter of her own plus a dozen foster children was dead. The cancer had spread to Georgia Montague's brain and she was bedridden for weeks before her death. Thomasine was by her side day and night. It was three o'clock on a September morning in 1975 when Georgia Montague died—her only daughter was holding her hand.

For almost two years afterward, Thomasine could barely bring herself to leave her house. The fear she'd felt since the day her mother was diagnosed—that she too would be stricken with breast cancer—intensified. Almost every night Thomasine would dream of her own death by breast cancer. "No one could convince me that I wasn't going to pass like she did. My mother and I shared so many things, we were so alike. I became more and more terrified of getting breast cancer. I'd sit on the couch reading and I'd be touching my breasts. I'd take three, four showers a day just so I could check my breasts."

Even when Thomasine put the fear aside and got on with her life—when she divorced her first husband and supported her son and two daughters and an adopted son by working on the assembly line in a shade factory and later as a clerical worker in a bank, when she remarried and was laid off from her job and suffered through back surgery and the death of her second husband from throat cancer, when hard times and continued back and leg problems landed her on social services—she worried about breast cancer and she waited. "All through the years, every day, I'd examine myself—feeling for the lump that I knew would show up one day."

She felt it on an autumn morning in 1989. She ignored the marble-sized lump in her right breast for two years and when she finally went to the doctor and had it removed, she was surprised and overjoyed to learn that it was benign. Still she didn't let down her guard. One year later, at the age of forty-nine, she felt another lump in the same breast. This time she didn't wait to get it checked. This time the diagnosis was different. Breast cancer.

As far as Thomasine was concerned it was a death sentence.

Her mastectomy last June revealed a three-and-a-half-centimeter tumor and ten cancerous lymph nodes. Surgery was followed by complications and immediate depression. Fluid seeped from her incision and the surrounding skin was burned and scaly. When the incision was drained, Thomasine was left with a

70

half-dollar-sized wound that was deep enough to stick almost an entire Q-tip in and that required daily cleaning by a visiting nurse.

Thomasine was about to turn fifty and that was a factor in her foreboding. "I saw myself walking in my mother's shoes. My mother died when she was fifty-two and my grandmother died when she was fifty-two—it was a heart attack—and I figured now it would be my turn. The cancer was eating me alive, I thought—and I fell to pieces. I didn't want to be around anyone. I stayed in bed and cried all day and all night. I was alone and doing too much thinking. I started to lose my faith in God. I was always told to pray—that no matter what, he hears you and he'll heal you. But he didn't hear me when I asked for my mother and if God didn't save my mother why would he save me?"

Thomasine's journey to recovery was a journey back to faith—faith in God, faith in herself and faith in the friends who shared her fears.

She'd phone the breast cancer hotline run by Adelphi University and cry to the volunteer who answered her calls. Finally she joined a support group, a decision that has paid off in survival for other victims. Studies show that breast cancer patients who join support groups survive about eighteen months longer than those who don't.

By this time she was bald from chemotherapy and enduring the headaches and nausea that came with it. But with the help of others fighting the same fight, Thomasine started to come out of herself. "I was the only black woman there but let me tell you, black or white, there's nothing like talking to another woman who has breast cancer because she knows what it's like to walk in your shoes."

Slowly, Thomasine tiptoed back into the world. The turning point came during a visit with her father in North Carolina. Thomasine went with him to his weekly prayer meeting, where the congregation had been praying for her since her diagnosis. As her father, Thomas Chavis, introduced her and said, "You've brought my girl a long ways with your prayers and now she's here with me," all Thomasine could think was, "Please don't let them ask me to say anything." They didn't but to her own surprise, Thomasine stood to speak. She told the roomful of strangers how breast cancer had shaken her faith and how she didn't think she could go through with her last chemo treatment when she returned home. "Please don't stop your prayers now because I still have a long ways to go," she said through her tears.

The meeting was a catharsis. "So many people out there were pulling for me, praying and believing in me, I thought maybe it was time I started believing in me too."

A few days later, when Thomasine was back in the pink-and-white house she shares with her youngest daughter, she went to her own church. When a parishioner asked, "Why haven't we seen you in so long?" a new Thomasine shot back: "Because I've been fighting a war, that's why."

And when she kept the appointment for her last chemo, Thomasine knew she'd really come a long way. The nurse asked Thomasine to talk to another breast cancer patient who was refusing to start chemotherapy because she dreaded wearing a wig. The woman didn't believe Thomasine's shoulder-length dark hair was a wig. So Thomasine proved it. I pulled it off and said, 'See. I'm still here—and I intend to be here for a long time.'"

Later that spring day—sixteen months shy of the fifty-second birthday that she still dreads—Thomasine Dembo stood at her mother's grave. She touched the white stone and whispered a prayer. And then she did what she always does—she placed a single white gladiolus, Georgia Montague's favorite flower, on the ground. But this particular visit was just hours after her last chemo injection and Thomasine didn't cry like she usually does. She stood in the spring sunshine and smiled and said out loud, "I'm not coming to you yet, mom. You'll have to wait awhile before you see me. I'm going to keep fighting. I'm going to keep living."

> *THOMASINE DEMBO: I had thick hair down past my breasts—with streaks of gold and red and silver in it like my mother's. After my second chemo, all I had to do was touch it and it fell out. It looked like I lived with twenty cats. I took a shower one morning and it's like all my hair melted off my head. I called my father in North Carolina and told him, "Daddy, we're twins now." He couldn't imagine it so I saved all my hair in a white plastic grocery bag to show him. I wore a wig to my support group and someone said, "Look at T, she hasn't even started losing her hair yet." So I said, "Oh, I haven't?" and I ripped off my wig and passed around my bag of hair. They were all amazed because there's enough hair in that bag for three heads. My daughter and her friends beg me to give it to them, or sell it, for hair extensions. But I say, "I don't care if it's not on my head, that's my hair and I'm keeping it." Sometimes when I'm alone I take the bag out of the closet and run my fingers through my hair. It still smells of shampoo. I guess one day it will grow back.*

CHAPTER 7

———

A Mother's Story

Liz LoRusso went right to bed when she came home from the biopsy that afternoon in October of 1989. Her husband held her until she fell asleep. "I needed someone to hold me," she would remember years later. "It's like I was a baby."

Her moment of dependency was a luxury. While she slept, Phil LoRusso went to the pharmacy to fill his wife's prescription and to the library to check out books on breast cancer. When he got back Liz was waiting on the couch—wondering what she'd tell her kids when they came home from school. There are few breaks from motherhood. Lauren was ten; Philip was six.

The minute Lauren LoRusso saw her parents, she knew something was wrong. "I figured it out from their faces. They looked scared. So I got scared."

They all sat together in the den—mother and father on the peach-colored couch, daughter and son on the matching love seat.

"We have bad news," Phil began.

"Mommy has breast cancer," Liz continued.

Lauren remembers the words that were spoken next. "My mom said, 'We don't know yet what's going to happen.' That made me more scared. I didn't know what it meant—what more could happen? I was scared, but I was young and stuff. I thought nothing bad could ever happen to my mom. She said, 'We're going to read books and talk to doctors, and mommy will get the best treatment possible.' She started to cry, then I started to cry."

Liz made two promises to her children. "I promise mommy will fight very hard to get better. And I promise I'll answer all your questions as honestly as I know how—I'll never lie to you about what's going on."

And Liz LoRusso never has. Not that it's ever been easy.

It wasn't easy that same night when a ten-year-old girl looked her mother in the eyes and whispered: "Will I get breast cancer, too?"

Liz had already done enough reading to know the odds. Liz LoRusso—who had no known risk factors for breast cancer—was about to rewrite her family history. She reached for her daughter's hand. "I don't know, Lauren," she said in a whisper of her own. "But because of mommy, you now have a fifty percent chance of getting breast cancer."

It wasn't easy a few weeks later when the children visited her in the hospital after her right breast and twenty-eight lymph nodes were removed. Only two nodes tested positive for cancer, but the tumor wasn't the usual concentrated mass. Liz' tumor was like an octopus—a malignant mass with far-reaching tentacles that measured almost eight-and-a-half centimeters. The children didn't know all these details when they walked into Liz' room at North Shore University Hospital, but they knew their mother had undergone a mastectomy. Liz had explained to them what that meant, but she wasn't sure they understood. Especially Philip, who'd announced to his first-grade class that his mother needed a wrist operation.

Lauren and Philip stared at their mother—pale and with intravenous tubes in her arm and gauze bandages visible underneath her pajama top. "I thought they'd run in and hug and kiss me. Instead there was this painful distance, this coldness." Liz broke the silence. She pulled her children closer. "Come sit with me on my bed," she said.

She put an arm around her son. "Where was mommy's operation, Philip?"

The freckled first-grader looked through his brown-framed glasses and pointed to his mother's wrist.

"Does mommy have a bandage on her wrist?"

The boy shook his head.

"Where does mommy have a bandage?"

Philip was silent.

Liz touched the bandages on her chest. "Mommy's operation was here, Philip. Mommy had her breast removed."

And it wasn't easy on the night when Liz tiptoed into her son's room to tuck him in. She stroked his hair and kissed his cheek. And a child whispered in the dark, "Mommy, how many times do you get breast cancer before you die?"

Liz still cries when she remembers that moment. "I was devastated," she says, "not for me, but for him. I'll never forget thinking—this sweet little boy is living with so much pain. My little boy is going to sleep every night wondering when his mommy is going to die."

Philip's mommy is still alive. She's still fighting breast cancer as hard as she can. And she's still trying to answer her children's questions as honestly as she knows how. She's still trying with love to make them understand about life and death.

Liz LoRusso, who is forty-one years old and who taught home economics for almost seventeen years, is still doing the job she's always wanted to do more than any other. The job of being a mother.

It was always that way. Ever since she was a freckle-faced girl watching the adventures of the Stone family on "The Donna Reed Show." She watched on a black-and-white TV in the living room of a house on a dead-end street in East Northport, a north shore community where potato fields had given way to high-ranches and split-levels. She was Elizabeth Marie Strohsnitter, the oldest of six children born within seven years, who shared a bedroom with her only sister and who went to mass on Sundays and taught baton twirling at Girl Scout camp in the summers. Alicia Strohsnitter was an at-home mom who wore high heels just like Donna Stone did. Norbert Strohsnitter was a Grumman engineer who went to work in a white shirt and tie and was home for supper with his family every night, just like Dr. Alex Stone.

It was the vision of family life that Liz carried with her into marriage. "I'd be mom in makeup and heels; my husband would come to the breakfast table in a suit and tie. My children would be polite and thoughtful and beautiful, and everything would be perfect."

On August 14, 1976, Elizabeth Marie Strohsnitter married Philip Michael LoRusso, who was starting his career in the world of business, a boy she'd known at Holy Family High School, who'd written in her yearbook six years before— "Too bad we didn't get to know each other better." They wanted children, so they bought a three-bedroom ranch—a government foreclosure with no electricity that they won with a bid of $36,650. Liz was teaching at a junior high and going to the state university at night for her master's degree; Phil commuted by train to his job as a controller in Manhattan. In their spare time they remodeled the kitchen and planted a lawn. They had a brand new bedroom set and a hand-me-down sofa that Liz reupholstered herself. Every Sunday after church Liz made a big pot of spaghetti sauce, and the Strohsnitters and the LoRussos all came over for dinner. Life was happy and uncomplicated.

By the time they'd transformed the ranch with no electricity into their dream house, Liz had her master's degree and she and Phil were about to become parents. "I was ecstatic," Liz recalls. "I was at the beginning of the generation of women who thought about not having kids. But not me—I was dying to be a mommy."

"I was terrified," Phil recalls. "I sat in the delivery room scared to death, because any minute my whole life was about to change."

And it did. But Liz didn't get to be Donna Reed at home in high heels. Lauren was born in December, and the following September the new mother was back in a classroom teaching high school.

By the time Lauren was a toddler, the LoRussos were at work on another fix-it-upper. Then, Liz' mother died suddenly of a heart attack. Four months later, her father was in a car accident that put him in the hospital for almost half a year. When he came home, it was to a bed in Liz' living room. A short time later, Philip was born.

And always, Liz LoRusso kept reaching for the dream that had beckoned to her from a television screen. If she couldn't be Donna Stone because real life didn't follow a script, she could still be the best mommy she knew how to be.

But on a September morning in 1989, something happened that the Stone family had never had to worry about. Liz LoRusso stood under a shower doing a breast self-exam—and she felt a lump in the upper inner quadrant of her right breast.

The night before the biopsy, Liz and her husband drove to a nearby park. They sat in the car and held each other.

"I want to see my children grow up," Liz said. "I want to be a grandmother. Phil, I don't want to die."

Even after the biopsy that told her what she didn't want to hear—Liz LoRusso kept on mothering. She wrote notes to her children's teachers, because, "hey, if my kid's not learning two plus two equals four, this could be the reason why."

And before she was admitted to North Shore Hospital on October 25 for a modified radical mastectomy, Liz made sure her son and daughter were ready for Halloween. Philip had a GI Joe camouflage suit from the Sears catalog. Lauren had a hand-sewn outfit that transformed her into a black cat. The day before surgery, Liz LoRusso baked twenty-four vanilla cupcakes for her son's first-grade party. She froze them, had the operation and five days later, she was back in her kitchen in the farm ranch-style house that she and her husband had bought from her father not long before his death. She sat with her right arm propped on a pillow and—with a little help from her mother-in-law—Liz LoRusso frosted the cupcakes.

By Christmas, Liz was in the throes of chemotherapy, and in different ways each member of her family went through it with her.

Liz would come home from her Wednesday chemo session and stay in bed until Sunday. Lauren and Philip would stand in the doorway and watch her sleep. Philip would sneak in and kiss her cheek. Sometimes, he'd sit on the bed next to her watching TV. His mother never stirred. Liz would go to mass on Sunday and for a ride with the family. By the time she was feeling stronger, it was time for another round of chemo.

"All I want for Christmas is my old life back," Lauren told her father as they decorated the tree that year.

He hugged her. "Don't we all."

The sense of family was like a magic lamp that shone through the long months of postoperative treatment. The chemotherapy lasted until June, and Liz' hair loss was traumatic for everybody. The oncologist had warned her that her hair would fall out within three weeks of starting the combination of chemo drugs known as CAF—Cytoxan, Adriamycin and 5-Fluorouracil or 5-FU. So Liz tried to prepare her family. She had her permed and frosted collar-length hair cut short, and she told her children: "Mommy's taking a lot of very strong medicine to try to get better. Pretty soon it's going to make mommy's hair fall out. I'd like you to help me pick out a wig. Would you do that for mommy?"

A few days later the whole family sat in a wig salon. Lauren took a positive approach. "Try on the blond one, mommy. Don't you want to be a redhead?" Philip watched silently from across the room. Every time Liz looked in the mirror, she wept.

Liz didn't wash her hair for six days because she dreaded being bald for the holidays. When she woke up the morning after Christmas, she knew it was time. She shampooed and when she came out of the shower she didn't even look in the mirror. She positioned one of her new wigs on her virtually bald head, then walked into the kitchen, where her husband and children were eating breakfast. She kept her head down to avoid seeing the reaction. No one said a word.

"I never knew people looked so different without hair," Lauren remembers. "She didn't look good. No one I knew had a bald mom. I thought maybe one day my dad could be bald, but I never expected to have a bald mom. When I had my friends over I didn't want her to wear a turban because you could tell she didn't have hair underneath. It was too weird. I made her wear her wig when my friends came over. I'd tell her, 'Don't you dare come out with a turban on.' I guess that wasn't too nice, but I was a little kid and I was embarrassed to have a bald mom."

They were all facing the realization that life is fragile and love doesn't conquer everything.

During the three months of radiation treatments that followed Liz' chemotherapy, her children met with an oncology social worker at North Shore. "Liz had a lot of sadness and depression—not just about her illness but because she was certain her children were hurting and she wasn't sure what to do about it," says Rosemarie Ampela. "Liz told me, 'I need help to make Lauren feel better.' Philip didn't seem to understand much, and in some secret part of Liz I think she was glad. Philip is avoidant; he denies—that's how he handles it.

"The most basic thing a child experiences when there's a problem in the family is—am I the cause? Kids feel responsible for crisis. Lauren and Philip were experiencing this guilt of responsibility. They'd also been fighting a lot. Most of it was sibling rivalry under stress. I reassured them that whatever was going on with their mom was beyond their control. I shared with them how surprised families— both parents and children—become when an illness enters. And that everyone handles these surprises differently.

"Liz began to understand that involving the children would be the key to everyone feeling better."

Every Monday morning during the summer of 1990, the mother and children would come to the hospital. While Liz was being bombarded with invisible rays of radiation, her children would draw pictures for Rosemarie Ampela. Pictures that told the story of a family in pain.

In one picture, eleven-year-old Lauren recreated in black ink the moment she learned her mother had cancer. Mother and daughter are sitting side by side on a couch, hands at their sides. The grown-up and the child are dressed alike; they both have dark hair. The mother is saying, "Lauren, mommy has cancer" as a tear rolls down her right cheek. The daughter responds, "Are you going to die?" and a tear falls down her left cheek.

The social worker saw a child's stress. "Lauren feels pressure to be like her mother—in her picture, they're the same size. This is an intensely emotional moment between mother and daughter. Lauren didn't feel that her dad and her brother were present at the time. It doesn't matter what the reality was, this picture shows Lauren's perception of the moment. There's tremendous pressure on the two of them—they're both crying. Mommy is crying in front of her, so she knows she isn't the only one with sadness and worry and fear. But their hands are down, not outstretched; they aren't touching, they aren't comforting each other. They each have a single tear coming out of opposite eyes—like they're a mirror image of each other, like they're sharing the pain. This mother and daughter stick together."

Philip drew a picture of his family. In almost a diagonal line across the paper, he sketched his dad at the top, a black figure with big hands and sticklike legs but no feet; his mom with lots of dark hair, and no hands or feet; his sister, towering over him; and himself—a boldly outlined cross-shape with no hands, no feet and no head. "I realized, wow, Philip sees himself as way down here," Rosemarie Ampela says. "Dad dominates. Mom is kind of helpless with no hands and no feet—so is Lauren. And then there's Philip. Poor Philip with no head—I don't want to know about this, I don't want to think, I don't want to feel, because I'm so helpless and so scared."

There were other pictures. Sketches of a sister kicking her younger brother. Sketches of a smiling girl in a shirt of chaotic colors, a reflection of her inner confusion, who promises "I will not fight with Philip"—and dots the i's of his name with purple hearts.

And a boy's picture of his family, with the caption—"When mommy's finished with her treatment, she'll probably be happy. She only has two more days to go. We might go on vacation if mommy feels o.k. and isn't pooped out!" The figures in the picture were labeled, "Dad, Lauren, Me." Liz wasn't in it. "Even if mommy is home, she's not there like she once was," Rosemarie Ampela says. "Philip missed his mother so much already, he forgot to draw her in."

But soon Liz LoRusso put herself back in the picture. "Liz didn't crumble in her role as a mother, and that's an incredible responsibility to maintain when you're fighting for your life," the social worker says. By April, 1991, the shadows were at bay. Liz was in the classroom again, and for two months life in the LoRusso household returned to the way it used to be. The way it was when Liz was a working mother who made time to bake apple pies and go to Little League games and teach her daughter's Girl Scout troop how to sew.

Then, in June, a routine bone scan showed cancer in Liz' spine.

Several months and dozens of tests later, Liz knew exactly what she was facing—the cancer had spread to her left pelvis and seven places in her spine. She had stage four breast cancer, the most advanced category, which according to established statistics meant she had a ten percent chance of surviving five years. By the time her children were starting school again, Liz was starting another round of chemotherapy—this time at Memorial Sloan-Kettering Cancer Center in Manhattan. It was an aggressive course of treatment in two phases—five months of outpatient care, followed by three months in the hospital. Throughout the treatment, there were complications—high fevers, hemorrhaging, renal failure.

During the outpatient phase, Liz fought to be a mom. When her family made their annual trip to the farms out east to pick pumpkins, Liz went along. She sat in a lawn chair, bundled up in a blanket, and watched her children romping through the fields. She went to Great Adventure amusement park and cheered at Philip's soccer games even though she'd broken out with such painful mouth sores from the chemo that all she could eat was Jell-O. Even her medication had to be pulverized. She lost her hair again. "Thirteen years ago I was petrified of becoming a father," Phil told her one night. "Now I face the possibility of raising our two children alone. Liz, where do I begin?"

Sometimes, her white blood count would fall so low and her temperature would climb so high that she'd be rushed to the emergency room at Sloan-Kettering. If it was the middle of the night, she'd leave notes on her children's pillows. "Mommy will be home as soon as she can. I miss you already. You're the best son a mommy could have and I love you very much." One night, she bent to kiss Philip goodbye, and his pain echoed in the dark. "I HATE WHEN THIS HAPPENS," he screamed. And then there was the time Liz opened her suitcase in her hospital room to find framed photos of her children that they'd slipped in her bag as a surprise. She still keeps those pictures by her bedside.

Lauren remembers one night in particular. "It was the first time I had to pack mom's suitcase. I was really scared. I remember telling Philip, 'Come on, we have to get mom ready; her fever is one hundred and four.' Dad was at a meeting at the yacht club, and Philip was playing Nintendo. I couldn't get him to stop playing Nintendo. So I packed mom's nightgowns and turbans and her little bag with toothpaste and stuff. I called my dad to come home and take her to the hospital and my grandparents to come over and stay with us."

During the inpatient phase of treatment, which started in January 1992, the mother could reach out only by phone. She tried to keep tabs on her children, she called to say goodnight—and she cried about the things she couldn't do for them. She cried when Lauren showed up at the hospital to model the dress her father had bought her to wear to a friend's bat mitzvah—a dark pink, off-the-shoulder, at-the-knee number that made her little girl look so grown up.

"How much?" the mother asked.

"It was on sale," the daughter said.

"One hundred and twenty-six dollars," the father answered sheepishly.

"Take it back."

"Mom, please. It's the nicest dress I ever had."

Lauren got to keep the dress, but Liz remembers thinking, "I wished I could have taken her shopping—that was my job. And I didn't know if I'd ever be able to take my daughter shopping again."

It was a long winter for the LoRusso family. After work, Phil LoRusso would visit his wife—he'd hold her hand and talk about the kids. By the time he'd board the 8:44 p.m. train to Huntington, where the LoRussos lived, his parents were driving the children home. Al and Jo LoRusso picked up the slack for their son: They brought the kids to their house after school, helped them with homework, fed them supper. Back in their own home, Lauren and Philip would curl up with their father on his bed and watch "M*A*S*H" and the "Tonight Show." Most nights they fell asleep with the TV on.

"Even when they were infants, Liz and I never allowed the kids in our bed," Phil says. "But somehow none of us had the energy to be alone. Maybe we were all just too scared to be alone."

"I liked sleeping in my mom's room," Lauren says. "We were all together, and I wasn't afraid or lonely. I felt safe there."

In March, Lauren and Philip put up a "Welcome Home" sign they'd made on their computer. Mom was coming out of the hospital. Her cancer was under control. She was frail; she used a walker. But it was springtime and Philip was playing for the Little League team and his mother attended every game. Summer bloomed and Liz was more mobile. She started another round of radiation treatments, she went on tamoxifen, but she also met the demands of suburban motherhood—shuttling her kids to wind-surfing lessons and soccer camp.

And as Liz LoRusso recovered her strength, her children saw a brand new mom. An activist mom, who joined a grass-roots advocacy group called "1 in 9," and wore buttons that said, "Silent No More!" A mom who carried placards and lobbied politicians.

A mom who made speeches.

"There is a war going on inside my body," Liz LoRusso told a rally last year. "To date I have fought and survived two battles, but not without many scars and struggles. In the last thirteen months my husband slept in our bed for ninety-one nights alone. There was no mother home to kiss the children good-bye before school. In addition, ninety-six days were spent arranging for child care, finding transportation and counting on someone else to take care of our children's needs, so that I could be in treatment. I've spent more days in treatment this year than my children have spent going to school. . . I want you to promise that you will not let up on your fight until this disease is known only to future generations in their history books. I don't want my daughter to have to hope for a miracle to see *her* children grow up."

Philip and Lauren had a mom who marched in Washington, D.C., during the National Breast Cancer Coalition's rally. Liz held aloft a cloth banner she'd sewn herself that proclaimed in pink capitals: WOMEN WITH BREAST CANCER ARE DYING FOR RESEARCH. She held it aloft with her husband and her in-laws and her aunt. And her children marched alongside her. Lauren and Philip carried a poster-sized photograph of some of their friends—four families with children, four families with mothers who have breast cancer. They attached a sign—WE WANT OUR MOMS TO LIVE!

"I was real proud of my mom that day," Lauren recalls. "I never saw my mom like that before. Everyone was yelling—'We want a cure. When do we want it? NOW. The wife you save may be your own'—but my mom, she yelled the loudest."

The march in Washington was the kickoff to summer. Liz was energized. When she came home, she had the kitchen remodeled. "I'm going to be a healthy mom in the kitchen again," she declared. And she decided it was time to have some fun. "This is my first summer in the past four that I'm not in toxic treat-

80

ment. This is a major event. This is going to be my summer of fun with the kids. I'm going to soak up love and laughter and good times."

She did. Even the simple moments were precious. Making fruit salad with Lauren for a teenagers' party. Buying Philip a New Jersey Devils cap. Eating pizza at Planet Hollywood. Chauffeuring the children to swimming lessons and to meet their newborn cousin in New Jersey. There were cruises on the family boat, *Philz Four Sum*, and a weeklong vacation at a resort upstate. There was the annual block party where the kids played relay races and Liz brought back her childhood with a hula-hoop.

There was the get-together with a group of friends at Jones Beach. Grown-ups sitting in the sand watching their children test the surf into the dusk. Sandwiches and ice cream. Hugs and laughter. And as the moon rose in a softening sky and the boardwalk lights glowed beneath it, Liz LoRusso shook out a blanket and stood looking at her kids and husband already ahead of her. For a moment, strain touched her face, and then she squared herself and strode forward in the sand.

There were other times when she had to square her shoulders at the summer. When an ear infection delayed her enrollment in an experimental course of immunotherapy in Chicago. When she found out the pain in her back was from three herniated discs—probably another side effect of vigorous treatment, like her arthritis and asthma. When she was told she'd have to wear a back brace and limit her driving and fit physical therapy into her schedule three times a week.

Now it's September. Soon the leaves will color the lawn of the house where Liz LoRusso dreamed of living like Donna Stone. The family will drive east to find the perfect pumpkin, and mom hopes to be in the fields and not on the sidelines. Life remains fragile for Liz LoRusso. She savors the seasons.

And as Liz deals with reality, the members of her family—each in their own way—deal with now and tomorrow.

Her husband shares her emotional pain. "I think Liz feels she got gypped. She may not see her children graduate high school. She's not going to see them graduate college. She's not going to become a grandmother. She's been gypped of all the things that mothers her age look forward to and take for granted. She's already lost so much precious time with her kids. We've all been gypped."

Her fourteen-year-old daughter tries to push away fear. "I try not to think about scary things. I don't know why, but sometimes grown-ups ask me, 'do I know that breast cancer is inherited?' I just roll my eyes and say, 'Oh geez, thanks for the hope.' Even when my mom was sick and bald and crying all the time, she was a good mom. I used to be afraid that maybe I wouldn't have a mom one day. But now, if I start to think like that or if I worry about her getting sick again, I call up a friend and talk about something happy. Or I watch a funny movie. I don't see the point of worrying about bad things that might not even happen. Mom's pretty much back to herself now—you better look out if you don't listen to her. But even when she yells at me I love her, and I know she loves me. I hope we have lots of time to argue with each other."

Liz' ten-year-old son holds his feelings in. Philip remembers when his mother's hair was "shorter than an eyelash," but he rarely says the words "breast cancer." He often tunes out when he hears them. Like the afternoon he breezed into his mother's room while she was looking through a bag of get-well cards she'd received in the hospital. Philip sat on the bed. "Mommy, can I have a friend over?"

Liz showed him a Valentine's Day card he'd made for her in the third grade. "Philip, do you remember this? You had all your classmates sign it, and you gave it to me in the hospital when I was so sick with breast cancer."

Philip looked at the cards strewn across the bed. He cleared a spot and rolled into a ball. He watched and he listened—but he didn't respond when Liz unfolded the welcome sign he'd helped string from tree to tree across the driveway when she finally came home. He sucked his thumb.

"Poor Philip," Liz whispered. "He doesn't like to remember; he doesn't like to hear. When he's confronted with it, he'll regress to a younger age. It's like he wants to be a baby, because babies need their mommies. If he doesn't grow up, his mommy can't possibly die."

Liz spent the next twenty minutes remembering the dark days. She remembered the time she came out of the hospital after a week-long emergency stay. "I went right to Philip's soccer game."

Suddenly, Philip came alive—"I scored fifteen goals last season," he announced. "It was my best season ever."

And, in an imperfect world, Liz LoRusso keeps working at the job she always wanted more than any other—motherhood.

"This is what happened to me in life, this is what my family was dealt. So what am I going to do, close the door and die while I'm still alive? Or live each day to the fullest. I tell my kids—when life hands you lemons, make lemonade. Breast cancer is a big lemon, let me tell you. But it's made me realize some things. I know now that high heels hurt and Donna Reed doesn't exist and who cares, because my imperfect family is perfect for me.

"I tell my kids what the doctors tell me—I'm treatable but not curable. I stress heavily that mom is doing OK right now and how no one knows what the future holds. I tell them I love them; I love being their mommy and I love being alive. I know it will take a miracle for me not to die of this disease—but I believe in miracles.

"And so with the Sword of Damocles hanging over my head, I'll live my life as completely as I can for as long as I can—and I'll keep trying to be the best mother I know how to be."

CHAPTER 8

Cindy Bluming: A Survivor

A year ago, Cindy Bluming had a double mastectomy—and an immediate reconstruction. "I didn't want to wake up without breasts," she says. "I wanted to wake up as close to normal as possible."

She woke to a world that would require a new definition of normal. There was nothing the surgeons could do about the deep and searing scars that breast cancer imprinted on her very self. The fear of death, the terror of the future.

"I'm wrestling with questions that seem to have no answers," Cindy Bluming says. "I'm not myself and I don't know if I ever will be again. Maybe someday as I get further away from it and remain recurrence-free. But right now I feel I'm a victim—a victim of breast cancer. It didn't just take my breasts—it took my core."

Actually, the core started disintegrating on Thanksgiving of 1992 when her best friend, Ellie Johnson—a colleague at the Locust Valley Junior-Senior High School where Cindy is a guidance counselor—was diagnosed with pancreatic cancer. Within six months, Ellie was dead—and Cindy Bluming had undergone a double mastectomy.

"We shared a love of gardening and reading and we shared the same birthday—August 17. Ellie, me and Mae West. 'The last of the redhot mamas,' we called ourselves. We were so alike, except that I'm Jewish and she was Catholic and I don't smoke and Ellie was a chimney. I gave her a gold cross for Christmas when she was in the hospital and she gave me a gold Star of David before my mastectomy. She reassured me that I'd be all right but as she got sicker I'd wonder, 'When will that be me? How long will it be before I'm lying in a bed—pallid with no hair and no dignity?' Ellie was so happy that she was around to see her granddaughter born. I started to worry, 'Will I live long enough to hold a grandchild in my arms?' I think my biggest fear is simply not being here anymore, ceasing to exist."

Cindy's fears were full-blown in February when she had a lumpectomy and learned that the cancer had invaded much of her right breast. A few weeks later, she underwent a mastectomy. And her left breast was so full of cysts that her surgeon recommended it be removed as a precaution. Like a lot of women, Cindy insisted on reconstructive surgery at the same time. "I'm very vain. I'm used to looking a certain way. I worried that if they cut off one I wouldn't match, that I'd look like a freak."

Two months later, when Cindy was in the throes of chemotherapy, her younger sister was diagnosed with breast cancer and underwent a lumpectomy. "I couldn't be the big sister for her. I was afraid to talk to her because I didn't want to bring her down." And then, just after Mother's Day, Ellie died. Cindy mourned for her friend and herself through the summer. In September, it was Rosh Hashanah, the Jewish New Year, a celebration of what had been and what was to be. And Cindy Bluming's core fell away a little more.

"I'm a Conservative Jew. I keep a kosher home. But I hadn't been to services in a long time. I wanted to go at Rosh Hashanah but I was afraid to hear the rabbi talk about the Book of Life, about who shall live and who shall die in the coming year. All I could think was, 'What am I looking forward to—more pain and sadness? Death?' I called the rabbi: 'Why do these things happen? I'm looking for answers. Where do I stand in the scheme of things?' Intellectually I know we all die but I thought I had plenty of time. My father is seventy-eight and he still rides a bicycle. But now I'm not so sure and I keep asking, 'What's it all about?'"

Questions without answers, days without reward. Cindy Bluming was used to being in charge. "I like to feel in control—even when I'm not." Before breast cancer, she thought of herself as Peter Pan. She was the mother of two grown children—Jason, a twenty-five-year-old computer engineer in California, and Diana, a twenty-two-year-old who works at the Whitney Museum in Manhattan. Cindy was a forty-nine-year-old woman who went to aerobics class four times a week. Now, all that seemed irrevocably lost. She'd sit alone and listen to Pavarotti and sob. "When I got breast cancer I lost control of my life. Even worse—I lost my innocence. I don't think I'll ever be carefree again."

Lost in her own fear and uncertainty, Cindy is trying to find her way back. But specters surround her. "I heard myself tell a student I was counseling, 'you won't always be unhappy.' I'm not sure she believed me. I'm not sure I believed me. In my work I'm surrounded by so much sadness. Two boys with moms going through bone marrow transplants, a girl whose mother died of breast cancer, four students who've lost their dads recently. I let the kids know I have cancer. Outwardly I try to present myself as a positive example."

Her husband, Sid, a lawyer, tries to help her. "I was always very driven professionally but now if Cindy needs me I take the day off without thinking twice. I'm more of a friend to her than I ever was. I feel helpless. It's hard to see the change in her personality. She was always the glass-is-half-full about life, always in control. Now she feels scared and weak and vulnerable—and not always for a visible reason. I react to her reactions—I'm saddened by her sadness. For both of us breast cancer was a life-altering event and we can't go back."

For Cindy and Sid, it made a difference that they were in therapy before breast cancer. And it helped that Cindy joined a support group when the counseling ended. "It's not that things weren't good," says Cindy, "but after twenty-seven years, we wanted to try to make them better."

Don-David Lusterman was the Blumings' psychologist. "It was nice serendipity that they were in therapy and had done a lot of work on their marriage before breast cancer arose," he says. "They were able to be more open and resilient with each other. She was honest about her fears and he was talking about his so they didn't feel isolated, they felt like pals. Sure, there's a part of this you have to face alone but if you can talk to your partner you're able to share that aloneness. Cindy's fears are appropriate—they need to be talked out, not pooh-poohed. She's not clinically depressed—she's functioning, she's respected in her work, she's in a healthy marriage. She's appropriately sad and vigilant and angry. There's a line from an e.e. cummings poem that goes something like, 'Always the beautiful answer . . . who asks the beautiful question.' Just asking those questions is, to some degree, part of recovery."

Cindy would like to believe that's true. "Life is a merry-go-round with lots of ups and downs but since breast cancer the downs seem to last longer. It's been harder to believe the ups will come around again. When I'm really down I don't believe they will.

"I keep worrying about the cancer coming back. I'm trying to get back in shape but I can't do the aerobics classes like I used to and I feel like a loser when I try. I resent the women I see working out, women who don't have breast cancer. I look at them and think, 'What did you have to deal with today, a broken nail?'"

Cindy tries and she makes concessions. "I'm facing the limitations breast cancer puts on my future. Getting a doctorate was my dream but I can't give up my salary and go to school full time and put that burden on my husband. Besides, I'm a lunatic and I wouldn't settle for anything but A's."

She searches for new definitions of normal. "My priorities have changed. I want to spend my time with my family. I want to learn French and play golf and travel and work in my garden. I want to marry off my children. I want to read more and brush up on my Hebrew. I'm thinking about getting bat mitzvahed.

"Sometimes I think, 'What right do I have to be unhappy?'" Cindy Bluming says. "How petty. But I'm sad. I weep for all I've lost—my breasts, my hair even though it grew back, my confidence, my optimism. I just ache. I worry about what I put my husband through and my children. Jason flew home to care for me and Diana drove me to every chemo appointment. She's convinced she'll get breast cancer and I can't help blaming myself for her fear. I'd like to put it all behind me but I can't. I'm not happy—then again I'm not dead either. Right now, I'm just not sure I'll ever be me again."

CINDY BLUMING: It's hard for me to accept help from others—I'm the helper. I'm used to being the one who brings everyone up. But now I'm the negative one. At every step it all turned from bad to worse. What was supposed to be a cyst turned out to be a malignant tumor. What was supposed to be a lumpectomy turned into a mastectomy; then one mastectomy became two. It rocked my self-confidence. It's like there's nothing to hold on to anymore. I've been stepping in shit all over the place and I'll never get out. I keep wondering what could I have done to prevent it? The answer is easy—nothing. It's all beyond my control.

————

Hermie Gibson: A Survivor

In 1972, when she had her mastectomy, Hermie Gibson knew only one woman who'd had her breast removed—a teacher in her son's elementary school in Great Neck. The woman came to visit while Hermie was convalescing. "It's not so bad," Hermie remembers her saying, "but you can never hang your pocketbook on that arm again. If you do it will blow up like a balloon."

It was a piece of advice her doctors had failed to convey about lymphedema, or swelling of the arm—a condition that once affected about twenty percent of mastectomy patients but now strikes only about five percent because less tissue is removed during surgery. And more than that, it was the first time since her operation that Hermie felt the relief of laughing with a woman friend. "I'd already cried enough to last a lifetime," she says.

The exchange of good advice and even better laughter was as close to a support group as a breast cancer patient could hope for two decades ago. Hermie would remember how nice it felt to know she wasn't alone. That's why she's been returning the favor ever since. For almost a quarter of a century, Hermie Gibson, the great-great-granddaughter of a slave, has not only survived breast cancer but she's been a good Samaritan for others stricken by the same disease.

Hermie's story of sharing and survival started the day she felt a lump on the top of her left breast. She thought it was a bruise because recently a box had dropped down from the top of a closet and hit her chest. She didn't go to a doctor for months and she might not have gone at all if she wasn't getting so tired—although some might say she had plenty of reason to be. She had five children at home ranging in age from eight to twenty-four and a husband who had pneumonia at the time, and she worked full-time as the director of a day-care center and part-time as a housekeeper.

When she finally went for an exam, the doctor sat down with her afterward. "She was a lady doctor and she broke it to me gently. She said, 'We're putting you in the hospital for a biopsy, and if we find that it's breast cancer, well, you won't have a breast when you wake up.'"

Hermie spent that night crying and praying. Her brother, who lived in Manhattan, brought a woman he knew who'd had a mastectomy to visit her. "She told me, 'Don't be frightened,'" Hermie remembers, "but I was." Then she underwent surgery and woke up with her fear confirmed by a bandage across her chest.

"When I came home I was withdrawn—even from my husband," she says. "I didn't talk about it. I'd cry when I was by myself."

But she had resources. She was glad to be alive and she leaned on her faith. "I prayed all the time. Breast cancer never shook my faith. I believed then and I still do that if I am to leave this earth or stay, it is God's will. As time went on I began to feel more sure that my time hadn't come. It helped when my doctor warned me about the weight I'd gained. He said, 'You're cured of breast cancer, but if you're not careful you're going to die of a heart attack.'"

And it helped that she had a friend who had gotten past the same fear. A friend who knew what it was to lose a breast to cancer. A friend who came to visit.

That's why Hermie Gibson—who had a radical mastectomy and twenty-seven radiation treatments, who wears a prosthesis and who can still be frightened by something as simple as a stomach pain—has made herself available to women she knew who had breast cancer. A few years after her mastectomy, a woman she had once worked for as a housekeeper was diagnosed. Hermie was there—shopping for groceries and cooking and taking care of her former employer's little girl. Hermie was there again when the woman needed a second mastectomy several years later. And she was there for the mother when the little girl grew up and died of the disease.

She was there for each of a half-dozen colleagues who worked at the school where Hermie is a teacher's assistant. She was there for Mona, who sat in the faculty room with Hermie one morning and cried when it was her turn to face the disease that her three sisters had already battled. Hermie put her arm around her crying friend and shepherded her into the restroom.

Months later, after Mona's straight hair grew in curly from chemotherapy, Hermie was stopping by her home every morning before school to share rolls and coffee. Then Mona was hospitalized and Hermie remembers a phone call. "I'm woozy," Mona said. "I'll talk to you in a few days." It would be nice if all of Hermie's acts of caring had happy endings. But breast cancer doesn't always work that way. In a few days Mona was dead.

Several years later, a teacher named Ruth was stricken. Ruth had been Hermie's youngest son's second-grade teacher—she had always invited young Steven into her house to see her aquarium. Steven now has a tropical fish aquarium of his own because of her influence. When Ruth came back to school, she asked to see Hermie's prosthesis. Once again, Hermie took a friend by the hand. "We were giggling like girls in the restroom," Hermie remembers. "Ruth told me it felt good to laugh and I knew just what she meant. She told me that because of me, she wasn't afraid."

But six months later Ruth was fighting a recurrence. The teachers asked Hermie to cook for the family on weekends because Ruth had raved about Hermie's cooking after she'd catered a faculty party. So Hermie spent every Friday in the kitchen—cooking veal roasts and pot roasts with all the trimmings, whipping up chocolate puddings and apple pies and strawberry tarts. Enough for Ruth and her husband and two children and her father who lived with them. And every Saturday morning for four months she delivered the meals to the family's home in Roslyn—and then she'd sit and visit with her bedridden friend. "Ruth always told me everything tasted even better because she knew it was cooked and packed with love."

One day, Ruth called Hermie into her bedroom. "She threw her arms around me and said, 'I love you so much.' That was the worst day for me. I could see her pain, I knew she was going to die. I told the teachers I couldn't handle going there anymore. I'd still cook but someone else would have to take the food to her. It was just too scary for me to see her."

Ruth died the following week. She was fifty years old and Hermie Gibson still cries when she talks about her friend.

Last summer Hermie bumped into a friend she hadn't talked to in a while—a pre-kindergarten teacher named Barbara Masry, with whom she'd worked on community projects through the years. Barbara Masry mentioned her latest venture—the establishment of the Great Neck Breast Cancer Coalition, a group that now has more than 100 members. Hermie Gibson signed on.

"Hermie said she'd had breast cancer years ago and she wanted to get involved," recalls Barbara Masry, who had a lumpectomy followed by chemotherapy and radiation treatments almost three years ago. "She's a real inspiration—because of her energy and enthusiasm and because having long-term survivors around boosts the morale of all of us."

As for herself, Hermie has annual checkups that include blood tests. But she refuses to have mammograms despite reassurances from her doctor that the amount of radiation is minuscule. "I don't want any radiation in my body," she says. So she does a self-exam every day of her life.

"I'd like to say I feel safe at this point, but who really knows?" Hermie Gibson says. "I'm not a brooder. I never thought about me too much. For me, helping other people is what it's all about. I never let breast cancer surround me—if you do that, it will swallow you up. I just take every day as a gift from God."

HERMIE GIBSON: I went into the operating room not knowing if I would wake up with a breast or not. When it was over, I kept thanking the doctors for saving my life. I was too happy to be alive to care too much about the breast. When they took off the bandage I was afraid to look. I thought there would be a big hole in my chest. I was relieved to see a straight line. I laughed when the doctor told me I could throw away my bra and join women's lib. I believe I've put breast cancer behind me. It's not always on my mind, it's just something I live with. But I can still be shaken. Three years ago my left arm swelled up and turned blood red and very hot. I'd had a cut on my finger and some of the children at school had strep throat and a germ invaded my body. Now I wear rubber gloves if there's even a tiny scratch on my hand. I even wear my watch on my right wrist.

Paula Leahy: A Survivor

Paula Leahy wore bright pink lipstick, L'Air du Temps perfume, a gold ring and a diamond ID bracelet to her lumpectomy. She had her nails done and she put her hair up in a French twist and brought along her favorite Michael Feinstein tapes for the surgeon to play in the operating room. Even when it comes to breast cancer, she does things her way.

Indomitable should be her middle name. Paula Louise Leahy stabbed her mammogram with a kitchen knife and cut out the tumor. She cursed her cancer and talked to her breast and nicknamed her radiation Rambo because she wanted to imagine a force powerful enough to annihilate her enemy.

And every day for the six years since her lumpectomy, fifty-three-year-old Paula Leahy has worn a pin above her left breast. She wears it in the exact spot where a malignant tumor once grew. She wears it as a medal of honor because she fought a war and, as far as she's concerned, she won.

Paula Leahy never even felt a lump. She got a clean bill of health at her annual gynecological exam in January of 1988. Three months later, her fingernails were cracked and splitting down the middle. "Something must be wrong with you," her manicurist said. "Go to a doctor." A few days later, Paula went to a holistic nutritionist in Manhattan, who found the lump and suggested a mammogram. "It was like when I met Donald, my husband. I knew in an instant that he was the man for me. I knew immediately that this lump was breast cancer."

She went to St. Patrick's Cathedral and lit a candle. "Dear God," she prayed, "please give me the courage to go through whatever I have to face with grace and dignity."

She didn't say a word to anyone—not even Donald Pirone, a mail carrier who was her live-in boyfriend at the time and who has since retired. "I had to get my head together, make a plan. I wanted to be alone with the tumor, the knowledge of it, so I could size it up, this formidable enemy I had to battle. I couldn't do that and take care of Donald so I sent him off on a fishing trip and I cried and drank a lot of red wine and prayed."

When she was alone, Paula Louise Leahy—who works as a customer service supervisor for Metropolitan Life—got down to business. She interviewed doctors, looking for a surgeon who, first and foremost, believed in lumpectomies and who would let her wear the gold bracelet with her name spelled in diamonds that Donald gave her on their first Christmas together and who'd play Michael Feinstein singing Gershwin and Porter and Berlin during the surgery.

Before Donald came home, she'd scheduled the operation. And she'd declared war on her cancer: "I yelled and swore at the tumor: 'I hate you, you fucking thing. How dare you invade my body, you s-o-b. I'm not going to let you ruin my life.' And I'd praise my breast, tell it how proud I was of it: 'You're so beautiful and brave. I promise I'm going to kill that horrible ugly tumor inside you.'"

And then on a Sunday, Donald returned from a week of fishing in Massachusetts. She made him sit on a white Italian porcelain foot stool in the living room. "I have something to tell you," she said calmly. "I have breast cancer."

Donald could barely speak as tears flowed down his face. It was the first time in seven years together that he'd cried in front of Paula. "Why you?" he asked. "You're so good."

"Why not me?"

"You don't deserve it. I had my whole future planned with you. It's not fair."

His words stung her. Paula remembers wondering, "How will he be there for me if he can't face it himself? How can I ever forgive him for being so selfish?"

"It's naive to think life is fair," she told him. "You'll have to take me to the hospital Wednesday."

They went out for pizza—"I was determined to make it a normal night," she says, "and in times of stress, we always run for cheese and tomato pizza and red wine." And as Paula Louise Leahy bit into the pizza, she realized what seemed to her a fundamental truth and turned philosopher. "I had breast cancer and the pizza still tasted like pizza. It was like a sign that life goes on. It was Donald's worst possible moment—I've never gotten over it but I'm crazy in love with him—and still the pizza tasted the same."

On May 12, 1988, the tumor—a three-centimeter malignant mass—was removed during a lumpectomy at St. Claire's Hospital and Health Center in Manhattan. When she got home later that same day, Paula grabbed a kitchen knife and attacked her mammogram. She cut out the tumor and threw it in the garbage can.

But she couldn't throw out her fear. She'd wake in the dark from nightmares. "I'd go, 'Donald. Donald. Wake up. Please tell me I'm not going to die.' After a few nights of that, all I had to do was call his name once and he'd click on like a tape recorder: 'You're going to live forever. You're going to live forever.' My darling came through in the end. I came home from the hospital with a drain hanging out of my left armpit and he'd gag when he had to empty it, but he emptied it. We called it the bucket of blood. He even washed me in the tub."

Two days after her lumpectomy Paula celebrated her forty-seventh birthday with a backyard barbecue and less than a week later she went back to work. She was a survivor and she decided she deserved her own decoration. So she wore her honor society pin from Suffolk Community College—she pinned it to her blouse just above her left breast where a five-inch scar stretches to her armpit. "I was so proud of my breast. It deserves a medal of honor." The next day she pinned on her mother's gold initialed locket which had been converted into a brooch and contains a photograph of her mother, Rita Stern, as a girl. And every day since then, Paula Leahy has worn a pin over her scar—from a polished brass angel Gabriel blowing his horn to a fourteen-karat lobster.

The summer after her surgery, Paula kept doing things her way. She refused to take chemotherapy.

"Two doctors insisted on it, two doctors said it wasn't necessary, so I did what I wanted." But she underwent seven weeks of radiation—better known as Rambo—and had what she calls the best summer of her life. "I was out on disability and Donald and I took our boat, *The Paula Louise*, to Fire Island for picnics. We cooked lobsters and steaks on the beach and I didn't get a single mosquito bite all summer."

After her radiation treatments ended, Paula went on tamoxifen—an estrogen-blocker that seems to be effective in controlling cancer. But even the routine of taking the little white pill etched with a woman's profile is strictly Paula Leahy. She makes it into a ceremony. Every morning, before she leaves for work, she places two pills in a miniature glass jar. She stands in front of the mirror and pins on her medal of the day. She reads a Bible verse and says a prayer and thinks about friends who've died of breast cancer. "Thank you God for today," she says. "I'm not going to waste it. And remember Joan—she was here and she's gone and I miss her." Then she takes one pill and leaves the other for after supper.

One year and one day after her lumpectomy—on May 13, 1989 —Paula Leahy and Donald Pirone celebrated her first anniversary from cancer with a victory. They got married. The blonde bride with a Boston accent wore a white tealength dress and lilacs in her hair, the silver-haired groom with blue eyes wore a white tuxedo jacket. They danced to "Through the Years" and toasted their guests in a garden ceremony—the friends who'd seen them through breast cancer.

She hasn't worn L'Air du Temps perfume since the day of her lumpectomy and she doesn't listen to Michael Feinstein anymore. And she's too nervous doing breast self-exams so she goes for checkups every three months.

But indomitable should still be Paula Louise Leahy's middle name.

"I'm living happily ever after," she says. "Breast cancer gives you the gift of freedom. I know now what makes me happy and I do it. I spend a fortune on books and music. I love movies and red wine. I've seen 'Phantom of the Opera' four times. I'm more selfish about my time with Donald. He's the best thing in my life and breast cancer gave me the courage to marry him. Breast cancer isn't the worst thing that's ever happened to me. I like to think that the worst thing that's ever happened to me hasn't happened yet. Cancer stinks but it can be a gift—you can learn from it and take some good from it.

"The thing is you can't let it control you. Breast cancer was part of my life. It's not my life. It didn't and doesn't own me. If it ever comes back I think I'll be able to handle it with grace and courage and dignity. But I can't waste today worrying about it. Because you know something, no matter what happens—the pizza still tastes the same."

> PAULA LEAHY: *You have to learn to say the word "Cancer—I have breast cancer." Sometimes you have to write it down time after time before you can say it. But once you can, that's the biggest victory—because if you can say, "I have breast cancer," you're halfway to saying, "I'm going to get rid of it." And finally, you can say, "I had breast cancer." You have to teach people to say it too. You can't settle for people saying, "'I heard you were sick.'" The insidious thing is breast cancer seems to hit women when they never felt better. Tell them, "No I wasn't sick, I only had cancer." Believe me it's good for a laugh. You see, women who've had breast cancer, you can't recognize them. We're just like you—standing next to you at work, in the supermarket, on the street. Yet we're not like you. Something happened that makes us different, incapable of smallness, not concerned over pettiness. Women who know how to laugh, how to live, who know how valuable every day is—rain or shine, who know that every moment counts. No, breast cancer shouldn't happen to a dog. God in his wisdom knew only women could survive it, live with it, conquer it—and be better for it.*

Epilogue

On a breezy spring Sunday, hundreds of men and women in the ballroom of a suburban hotel looked up from their scrambled eggs and fruit salad at the teenager on the podium. The teenager's long dark hair framed a face that seemed forever solemn. The teenager's eyes were dry but her voice trembled and it matched the tears glistening in the eyes of her aunts and grandmother who sat in front of her. The teenager's name was Lauren LoRosso and she was describing what it's like when your mother has breast cancer.

The tears gathered in my own eyes, too. Earlier I had walked around the room greeting oncologists and social workers and activists I had gotten to know over the past year and a half, and embracing women who had left their imprints on my life. I hugged Francene Montalbano and Daphne Jackson and Thomasine Dembo. They looked beautiful. So did most of the other people in the room—men and women who were celebrating the simple and overwhelming fact of being there. It was the American Cancer Society's annual Survivors Day Breakfast. Lauren LoRusso and Francene Montalbano were among the guest speakers.

Francene told her story—the story of a woman's journey to hell and beyond and back again. She told it with indignation and disbelief but she also told it with humor and exuberance. Six months later she and Jaime would spend their happiest Christmas together—and she bought him a little blue van and four train sets and it took the two-year-old a couple of days to open all his presents. And then shortly after Christmas, Francene was hospitalized with a viral infection that was a complication of her cancer. The new year had barely begun when she died. "Fran tried so hard, she just kept trying and trying," said her sister, Rosemary Cottone. "She was just starting to feel happy again and to plan a life again."

But on that spring Sunday in a hotel ballroom the future was far away. On that spring Sunday Francene Montalbano was clearly a survivor as well as a victim.

So, in her way, was Lauren LoRusso, who like most fifteen-year-old girls, worried about grades and boyfriends and whether she should try out for the kick team, but who also worried about whether she would get breast cancer. And who on this breezy spring day had to be frightened for her mother. Liz LoRusso was back in the hospital—fighting an infection caused by the illness that hovered over her family. The illness that would hover over her family for another seven months—until January 19, 1995 when Liz LoRusso died of congestive heart failure, a complication of the advancing cancer. Lauren's theme was that when it comes to breast cancer, children are victims, too. So are husbands and parents and friends and relatives. When it comes to breast cancer, we're all in it together.

We're all in it for good and for bad and for always. That's one of the basic precepts Erica Berger and I learned from an assignment that bordered on a lifestyle. For almost two years, we lived other people's lives. We shared Marc Rosenbaum's grief as the hospital bed his wife would no longer use was removed from his home, we smiled in the glow of Fran and Jerry Lenzo's second honeymoon, we sat in the half-light of dusk at Jones Beach and watched Liz LoRusso watch her son scramble in the waves. We learned that in death as in life, no one should be alone. The support groups of breast cancer extend beyond meeting halls into all the rooms of our lives. We're all vulnerable. Maybe that's where caring starts.

From early on, this was a constant object lesson. This is not the venue for an exercise in self-revelation but it's pertinent that both Erica and I come from backgrounds where people tend to hole up in their own private hells. I think Erica explains it best. She postponed college to stay with her dying father, but they hardly ever connected. They needed each other's reassurance and didn't know how to give it. During the breast cancer assignment, Erica's mother had a heart attack. Erica was more involved in her care than she had been in that of her father. She attributes this to what she learned from watching the Rosenbaums and the LoRussos cope with cancer. As for me, last Christmas the packages I gave my adult stepdaughters and my sister and my mother included exam cards like the one that still hangs in my shower.

We also received lessons in courage—the quiet courage that sings through the personal and at the same time epic dramas of everyday life. The kind of courage it took for Liz LoRusso to arrange her daughter's surprise sweet-16 celebration just one month before Liz's death. She made the plans from her hospital bed at Memorial Sloan-Kettering, booking tickets to the Broadway musical "Crazy for You" and arranging for a stretch limo to and from the theater. And then Liz made sure she was released from the hospital. "I want to see my girl's face as she watches her first Broadway play," she told me when I visited a few days before the big surprise.

The kind of courage it took for Edith Kmetz to lift her husband from his wheelchair to their bed on the same night she came home from having her breast removed. The kind of courage it took for Lorraine Timmes to live on oatmeal and milk because of the mouth sores caused by her chemotherapy. The kind of courage it took for Thomasine Dembo to beat back the phantom of her mother's death from the same disease she now faced.

And the kind of courage it took for Sue Rosenbaum to go on living as she lay dying. Sue lives in all of us. Three months after Sue's death, her daughter Naomi got married. Baby Alexis was there, and Marc and Jesse. The guests talked about Sue, about how happy she would have been. And just a few weeks ago, I happened to be in Long Beach. I drove by the esplanade that runs in front of the house where Sue lived. It was fall and chrysanthemums bloomed crimson and white on the cooling earth. A picnic table with a wooden canopy stood at one end of the flower bed and a sign stood at the other. The sign is an official marker erected by the city. A proclamation honoring the human spirit. "Sue's Garden," it reads.

There's one other thing. I've always been a lone wolf in the way I work. This time it was different. Erica Berger and I had never worked together before.

94

We started the assignment as colleagues, we finished as friends. And part of our friendship will always be the shared experience of entering the lives of brave and wonderful women and coming out with the words and the photographs we have presented here.

Irene Virag
Long Island
January 1995

WHAT SHOULD I DO?

A woman's chances of surviving breast cancer depend on early diagnosis and treatment. The only thing you can do is get screened regularly.

The American Cancer Society guidelines for screening are:

- At age 20: Get a physical breast exam every three years and do monthly self-exams.
- At age 40: Do monthly self-exams, get an annual breast exam and a mammogram every year or every other year. After a year of debate, the National Cancer Institute recently stopped recommending routine mammograms for women under 50 based on studies that failed to show they save lives. But the cancer society, and many doctors, continue to recommend them.
- At age 50 and up: Do regular self-exams, get a breast exam and a mammogram every year.

If you have any relatives who had breast cancer at young ages, counselors advise starting regular screening even earlier than 40. This is something to discuss with your doctor.

The National Cancer Institute operates a toll-free hotline, (800) 4CANCER, which provides up-to-date information on breast cancer prevention and treatment.

ABOUT THE AUTHOR AND PHOTOGRAPHER

Irene Virag is a Pulitzer Prize-winning reporter for *Newsday*, where she writes the "Long Island Diary" column. A native of Bridgeport, Connecticut, she studied literature at the University of London and holds a bachelor's degree from Boston University and a master's from the Medill School of Journalism at Northwestern University. She was awarded a Nieman fellowship at Harvard University and has won numerous writing awards. She lives on Long Island with her husband, Harvey Aronson, a novelist and *Newsday* editor.

Erica Berger is a native of Miami and a graduate of the University of Florida. A staff photographer at the *Miami Herald* before joining the staff of *New York Newsday*, she has been nominated three times for the Pulitzer Prize for feature photography and has exhibited work in New York City galleries. She has won the national Society of Professional Journalism award for deadline photography and the University of Missouri Pictures of the Year award.